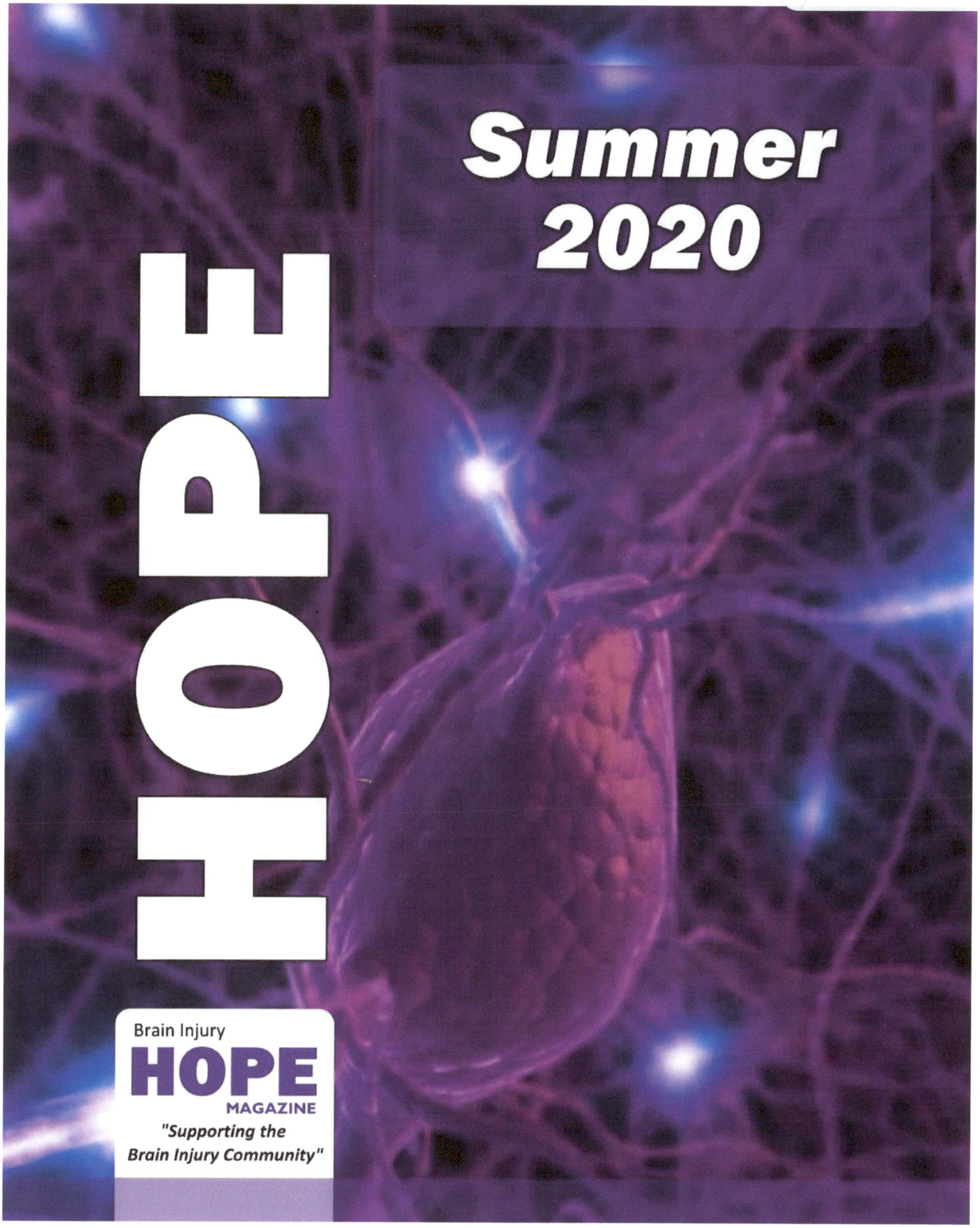

Summer 2020

HOPE

Brain Injury
HOPE
MAGAZINE
"Supporting the Brain Injury Community"

Welcome

HOPE MAGAZINE

Serving the Brain Injury Community Since 2015

Summer 2020

Publisher
David A. Grant

Editor
Sarah Grant

Our Contributors
Patrick Brigham
Lethan Candlish
Donna Cramer
Jeanette Drake
James Martin
Natalie McDonald
Alonso Mendez
Carol Nickerson-Goguen
Isaac Peterson
James Scott
Jeff Sebell

Welcome to the Summer 2020 Issue of HOPE Magazine

Little could any of us have foreseen the changes that have come to pass since our last issue was released in early March. A pandemic has affected people all around the globe. Most traditional brain injury support groups have been cancelled out of an abundance of caution. Many have moved to virtual meeting platforms like Zoom, while others have simply closed their doors.

Brain injury conferences have been cancelled around the world, and with that, the loss of sharing life-changing information in a face-to-face environment. Waves of protestations about racial inequality justifiably fill the evening news, offering hope that we may actually be on the cusp of long-overdue meaningful societal change.

In the midst of this all, it remains our hope to be a source of familiarity, comfort, and perhaps inspiration to those who are struggling today in ways they never envisioned.

Be safe and be kind.

Peace,

David A. Grant
Publisher

Table of Contents

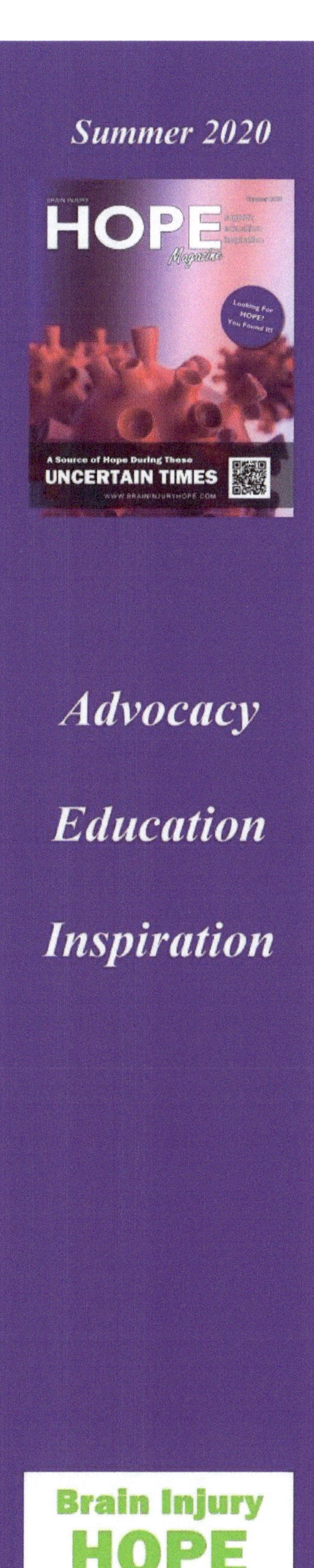

Got a Headache?

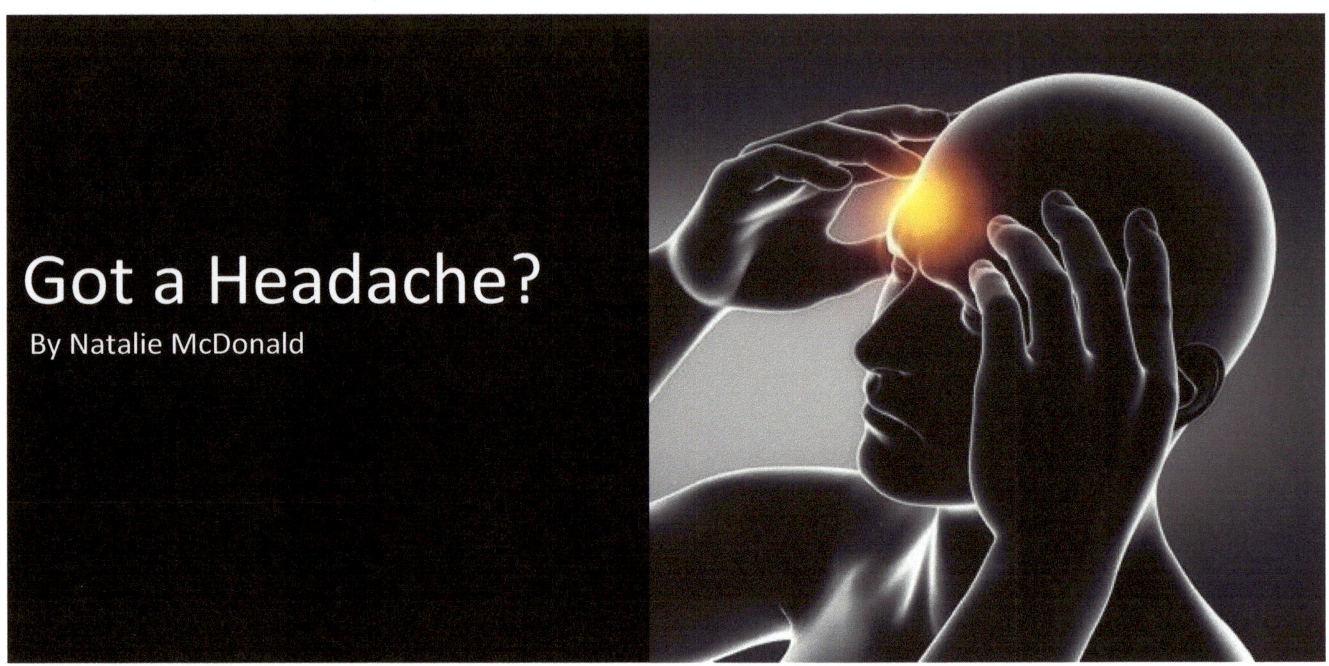

By Natalie McDonald

"I'm sorry, I'm not angry with you. My head just hurts." My son was eating dinner with us that evening and had asked me a question. I had been trying to answer him and had gotten confused and pretty irritable. And my voice was rough-edged, as it is too often these days.

I apologized, and he replied, "It's okay, Mom." Then he said-only semi-jokingly, "Mom, when DOESN'T your head hurt?"

When I go to support group meetings or read articles, the subject of TBI headaches always comes up. This makes sense, after all, what is a traumatic brain injury? In plain English, it means that you hit your head hard. It doesn't take a genius to figure out that would result in some head pain.

But wouldn't it be cool as if in cartoons, you just got a big lump on your head, your eyes went round and round, birds would circle your head for a few seconds, and then in the next frame everything was back to normal? Don't we wish! But sadly, it's not. In real life you have to deal with trips to emergency rooms, hospital and medical personnel, all sorts of endless paperwork, and all sorts of other complexities.

I never had migraines before my TBI. But there is no getting around the fact that after a brain injury, these headaches are far more common, often seemingly more intense, and the issues around how to treat them are often more complicated.

> "When I go to support group meetings or read articles, the subject of TBI headaches always comes up. This makes sense, after all, what is a traumatic brain injury?"

The question is how to deal with brain injury headaches. No two people will find success with the exact same methods, because there are all manner of headaches after a brain injury. No two injuries are the same and no two people are the same. There is an infinite complexity of variations.

My particular brain injury was a severe, closed-head TBI caused by a car wreck. I was in a coma for two months, then slowly came out of it. I had lots of internal injuries, but the most relevant to my ongoing headaches was my all-over brain damage and my severe neck injuries. I am home now, living with my husband, but was unable to resume my former career as a vocal teacher/church music director. I am able to spend most of my days in relative quiet and peace. I tell myself this is fortunate, given my need for rest and silence now, as well as my relative inability to complete tasks.

We never watched much television, but music was a constant in our home. That is no longer the case. I believe this is one big reason for my headaches being more manageable now. I keep busy with household tasks, stopping to rest frequently. I am extremely fortunate to have a husband who is still able to work outside the home.

I need to monitor my own health closely now. This is very annoying but quite necessary. At least I am far more able to do this than I was in the past, which is a huge celebration for me and, I am sure, for my long-suffering family. I do really try to fend off the headaches as much as possible.

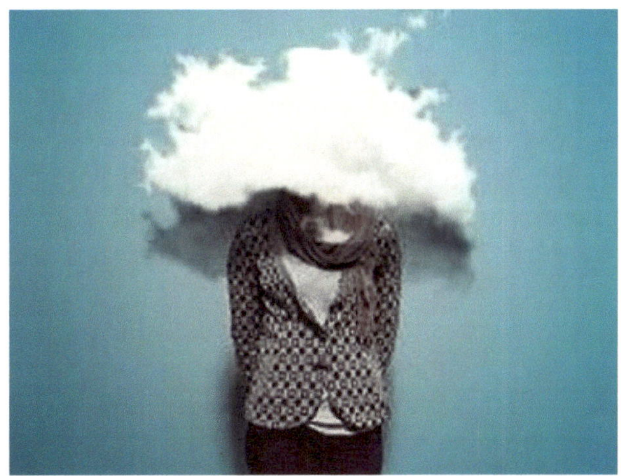

Once the dreaded head pain starts, things quickly get much worse. The mental fog thickens, and I get increasingly clumsy. I feel stupid and thick-tongued. My body temperature goes rapidly back and forth between too hot and too cold and random aches and pains appear elsewhere. My mental processing speed slows almost to a complete stop. I sometimes stare, not taking anything in, then start to shake. My sudden surges of anger makes me feel like Mr. Hyde.

There is plenty of incentive to try to prevent, or at least lessen, my headaches. While not intended to take the place of any medical advice, here are a few suggestions that I have found to be effective for me.

1. Plan ahead. Pain is much easier to prevent than to stop once it has dug its claws into you. If my plans include some possible headache triggers like conversations, music, too much thinking, hormonal stuff, etc., I take a couple of ibuprofens or acetaminophens beforehand. You may have some prescribed pills for this purpose. I do my best not to overuse these, as the threat of rebound headaches is always present.

2. Stay loose and keep relaxed as much as possible. I pause to take deep breaths and stretch frequently throughout my days. Peppermint oil and unscented body cream, mixed together, make a great massage cream for the neck. Periodically I do stretches throughout the day because I hold myself so abnormally now.

3. **Peppermint oil.** As mentioned above, peppermint oil I find to be an essential item. When I feel a headache coming on, if it's not an "icepick" or a "sledgehammer" one that requires instant medication, I dab the oil on some or all of the following spots: temples, behind and front of ears, jawline, under my nose, my "third eye," and sometimes a little on my tense neck muscles,

 4. **Ice packs.** I use ice packs across my temples or on the back of my neck. Sometimes, when the pain is severe, I immerse my feet in hot/warm water at the same time.

5. **Yoga.** I can't drive myself and we're on a tight budget, so it's tough finding classes. I have found great options on YouTube. This has been immeasurably helpful in aiding me through my recovery. I am far more flexible, at peace, and pain-free these days than I would have been without it.

6. **Staying in shape and monitoring my diet.** This is annoying advice because we hear it all the time, but it does really help with headaches also. Instead of a mindset of "I can't eat that" I try to think of what I can eat, and then keep plenty of those foods around. Infused waters in attractive containers, encourage me to stay well hydrated.

Keep persevering until you find solutions that work for you. I understand it can be very frustrating. I have been four years on twice-a-day migraine pills, which fortunately seems to fend off most of my headaches. I only need supplemental ibuprofen or acetaminophen, or one of these other remedies, every few days now.

I have also learned, on days when the pain just will not go away, to "lean into" the pain and try to stop being afraid. I have found that fear of hurting is often worse than the pain itself. I enter into the headache and just try to calmly have a look around, without being angry at it. While I'm in there, I pray and meditate. Sometimes it helps to think clinically about the bodily process that is happening that results in my headache.

Sometimes, I cannot think this hard. I just try to think of things *like, "I suppose I'm grateful to at least I have a head that hurts right now."* When it is hurting extremely horribly, I imagine a whole silly movie reel in my mind of someone chopping my head off with a guillotine, and then putting it in a basket with a bunch of other heads. I seem to be sufficiently amused by that to get a little relief. Because sometimes, frankly, I hate my head.

Most of the time, however, I am just grateful for the blessings of modern medicine and, for most of us, our ability to live a healthier life. Here's wishing all of us headache free days - or, at the very least, bearable headaches!

Meet Natalie McDonald

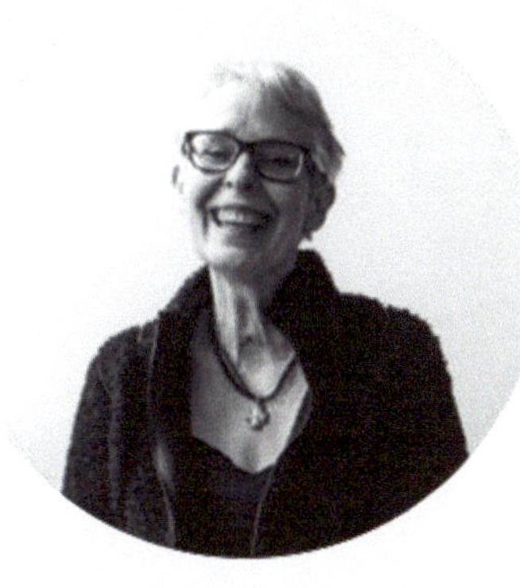

Natalie McDonald lives with her husband Marty outside of Des Moines, Iowa. They have four adult children, Alanna, Ali, Nate, and Evan, and two amazing granddaughters. Natalie suffered a TBI in a car crash in Sept 2014 on her way to an evening musical rehearsal. She was in level 1 coma for 2 months: she was first in ICU then transferred to another section of the hospital. Before Thanksgiving she was taken to On With Life, a brain injury rehabilitation center in Ankeny, IA.

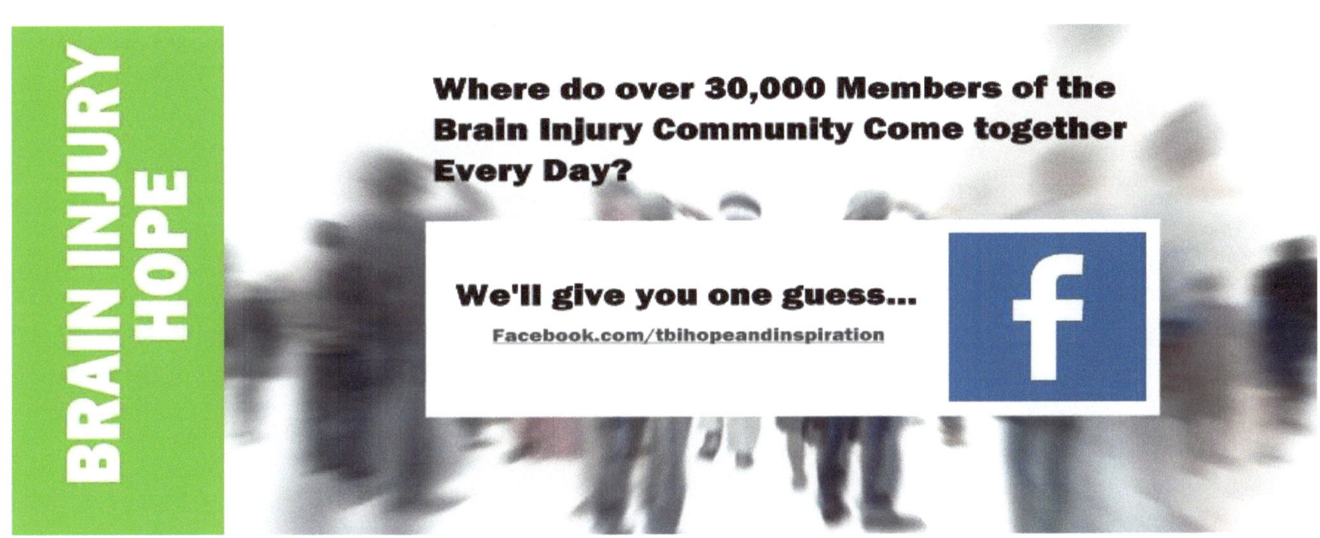

Chattering Monkeys

By Jeff Sebell

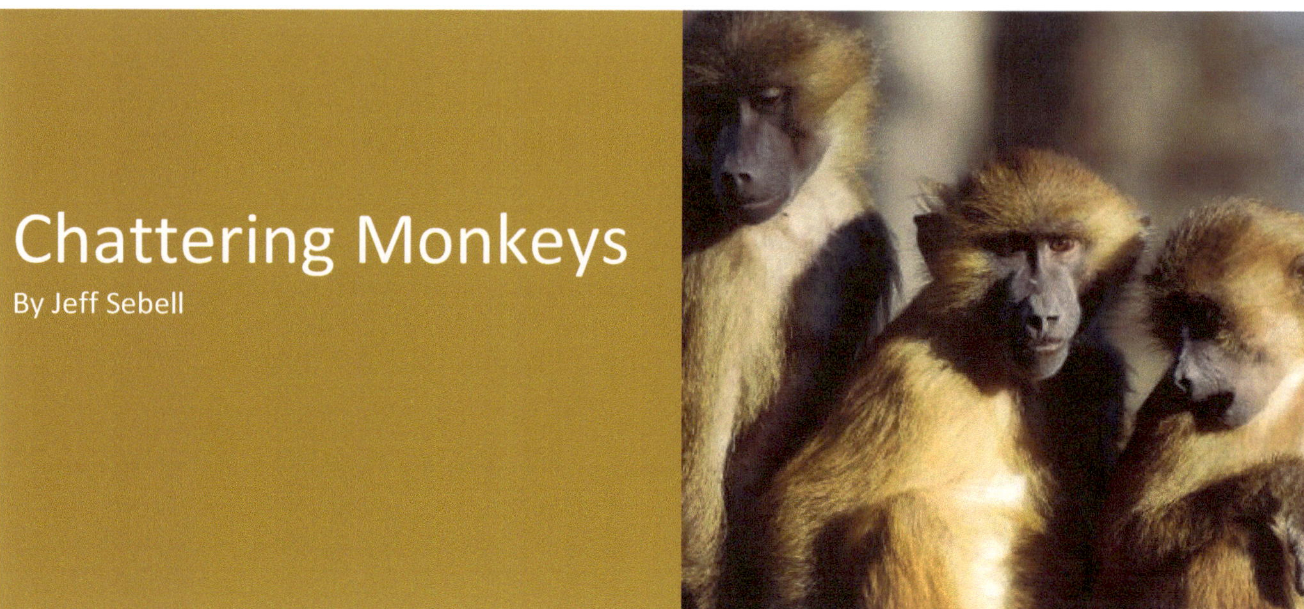

You know what I'm talking about: the crazy, never-ending noise in our heads; questioning, debating, not believing, not trusting.

The bedlam in our brains. That infernal, mind blowing racket that stops us in our tracks.

Now, this noise may not begin immediately, but after the initial shock and trauma of our brain injury begins to wear off and we start looking for our old lives, that noise comes out in all its glory, telling us that we can't do this or are unable to do that, that we are no good. Our heads are filled with crippling doubt and anxiety. We come to grips with the idea that we are never going to be what we once were, and that we cannot do anything right. Our future looks like a big black hole, and we worry about what will become of us.

> "We come to grips with the idea that we are never going to be what we once were, and that we can't do anything right."

While its true that those of us who have experienced a brain injury can have any number of serious physical or cognitive issues, the noise in our heads; the emotional and mental effects of brain injury, can be the most debilitating and difficult to live with.

We all do our best to work around any physical and cognitive issues, but these mental and emotional issues are hard to deal with. They prevent us from reaching our potential and they take away the ability to live our lives. They make us feel helpless; we cannot explain them or understand them, and we do not know what to do about them. We just accept their relentless roar in our heads as one of the consequences of brain injury.

What To Do?

Some of us we think the noise will go away when we find a way to "fix" ourselves and get back to the way we used to be. Others decide to see a social worker or a psychiatrist, trying to find answers.

Personally, I found myself unable to do anything about what was going on in my head; the constant jibber jabber that rolled around in my brain as I went about my daily life, making me miserable, making me not care if I lived or died.

I did not understand the doubt, lack of confidence and the questioning, and I reluctantly accepted them as something that was always going to be there until I "got better" someday. I also learned to accept my situation, along with my depression and my loneliness, as though it was a fate I "deserved".

My thoughts were out of control, and I could not do anything right. I found myself trapped. I longed for the way things used to be, back when my mind worked for me and not against me.

By itself, all this noise was hard to live with, but there was something else: the noise made me constantly worry. I worried about what I thought. I worried about what other people thought. I worried about what other people thought about me. I worried about my future. I worried about my present. I saw no way out.

I drove myself crazy this way and, in my mind, I became an insignificant person in the world: a person without any value.

A Way Out?

I needed help; someone to point me in the right direction. Then I discovered something Buddha said.

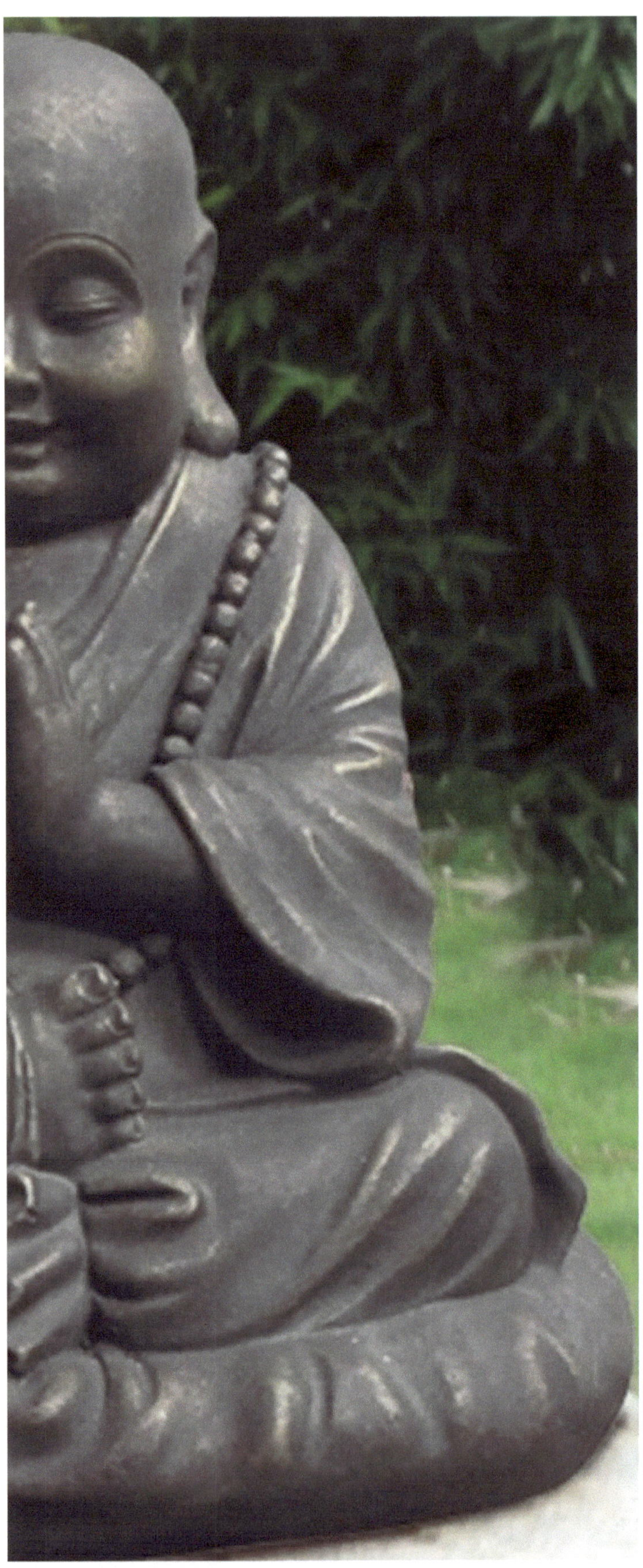

Buddha talked about how each person's mind was inhabited by chattering, or drunken, monkeys. These monkeys would swing from tree to tree, high in the jungle of our minds, screeching and laughing. The noise of these drunken monkeys was so loud that we would become paralyzed; caught up in how bad the chattering made us feel.

When I heard that, I saw a light, and maybe a way out. Finally, Buddha had given me a name for all that racket; for my affliction. l had a name for all that noise, and maybe now I could figure out what to do about it.

Come, Sit Down and Make Yourself Comfortable

I could not come up with a way to simply rid myself of the monkeys; they were just too ingrained, but what Buddha helped me with was finding a way to accept and tame those monkeys so I could live with them. I had taken the first step; understanding the existence of the monkeys, but what do I do next?

The solution sounds strange, but it is this: forget about what the monkeys are "doing to you" and learn to focus, instead, on making them your friend. Sounds crazy, but if you begin by accepting them and understanding that they aren't going to go away, you can make some headway.

Let's face it, these monkeys are your neighbors, and it always works much better when you get along with your neighbors - even when they don't make your life easy. Work to have your mind be a positive force by going out of your way to accept and talk to them; have a conversation with them.

Be calm. Acknowledge the monkeys and engage them in a way that helps you.

Learn to talk to them, become familiar with them. Tell them you know what their game is and make them your friend. Each emotion has their own monkey, and you can even give them all names. Fred the fear monkey. Alice the anxiety monkey.

When we have had a brain injury, our well-being is not only affected by what happened to us, but it is also dependent on how we choose to approach life after our injury; on the choices we make. We want to live the best life we can, regardless of how our brain injury has impacted our lives, so we have to put our best foot forward by finding different ways to make our lives work. One way we can do that is by making an effort to live with the monkeys.

Make the choice to have your mind work for you. Engage the monkeys. Tell them you are happy to see them and ask how their day has been. Tell them you know what their game is. Tell them, "That was a good try, but I'm not falling for it this time." Learn to speak up for yourself, not with fear, anger or by being confrontational, but with the truth, sincerity and strength.

When those negative, chattering monkeys come a-calling, stop for a second and think about what those voices really are and remember the power in you…the power to understand and live the life you want and not be trapped by what the monkeys say.

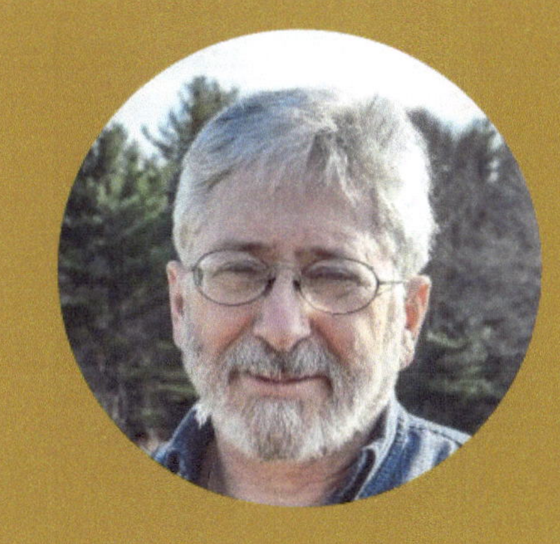

Meet Jeff Sebell

Jeff Sebell is a published Author, Speaker and Blogger writing about Traumatic Brain Injury and the impacts of his own TBI which he suffered in 1975 while attending Bowdoin College He has been active in the community since the inception of the NHIF, and was on the founding board of directors of the MA chapter. His book "Learning to Live with Yourself after Brain Injury", was released in August of 2014.

Hope is being able to see that there is light despite all of the darkness.

~Desmond Tutu

My Journey

By Donna Cramer

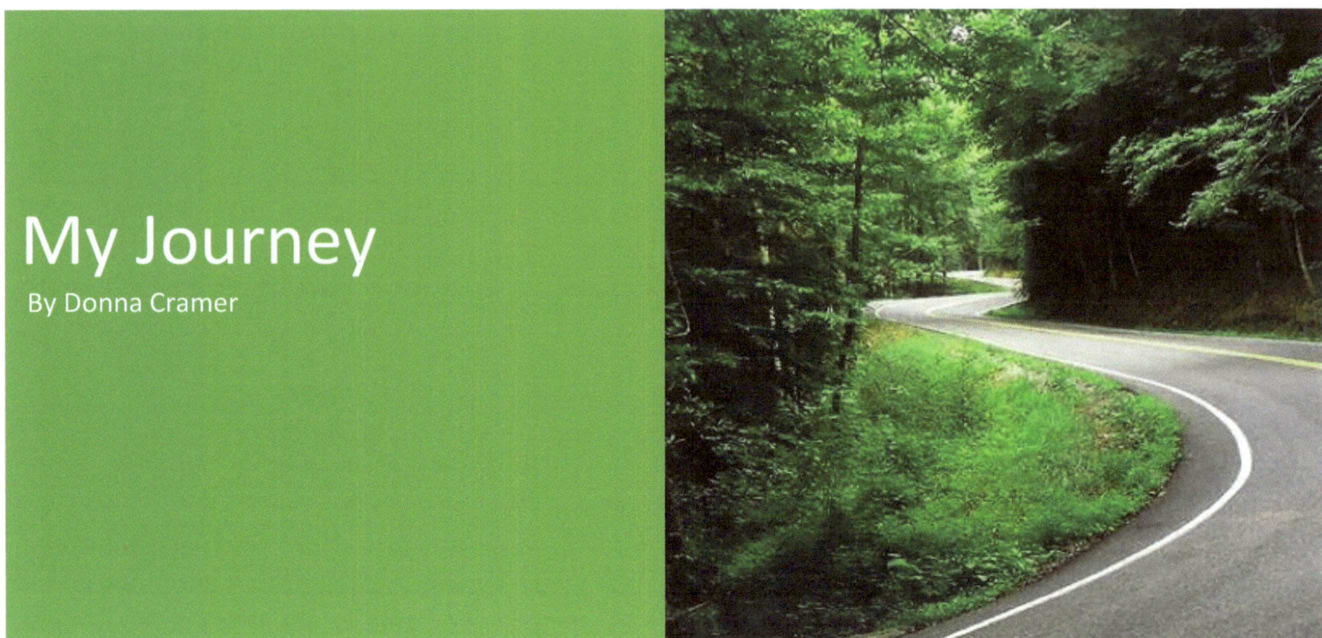

I am going to start at the end of this story instead of the beginning. The beginning is too hard. My husband went to school today. I was a teacher. He picked up all my belongings. They were on a cart in the hallway. My life for twenty years was on a cart in the hallway. Twenty years packed into a few boxes does not look like much.

I have been on a long, extended journey that I did not choose to go on and certainly never dreamed that I would take. I have not been in my classroom for four years. Someday I will accept the fact that I am never going back. I know I am never going back because today I received a letter in the mail granting me disability retirement. What a long, strange torturous trip it has been.

> *"I have been on a long, extended journey that I didn't choose to go on and certainly never dreamed that I would take."*

I worked with special needs students in a combined age classroom preschool through first grade. My students were autistic and non-verbal. Life was hard for them. The first incident happened when I attempted to help my assistant calm one of the students. I leaned in front of his chair just as he kicked his feet out. He was strong and, on my haunches, I fell back. I bumped the back of my head. It hurt, but I thought it was no big deal.

Lesson #1: Small hits to the head can cause damage. Every head injury should be checked out. My youngest guy comes in distraught the next day. He is crying. I have him on my lap and am rocking gently to quiet his pain. I am also looking around the room trying to monitor the others. I am watching a boy prone to violent outbursts, and I also need to monitor the boy who was removed from his home and is now in foster care because any violence triggers strong PTSD reactions in him and can trigger violent outbursts of his own. As I look around the room, the boy on my lap stiffens his body and gives me a hard-backwards head butt directly to the forehead. I see stars and feel I might pass out. I am urged to go to the nurse, but I decline there is too much going on in the room.

Lesson #2:   You do not have to pass out to have sustained a severe injury. Head injuries can be life-changing. I have a terrible headache which I attribute to stress, and I feel dizzy driving home, which I attribute to the heat. It is late August. My husband says that I acted differently that night. I remember very little of that night. The next morning, I am dizzy, and both light and noise sensitive. I have a banging headache. One of my boys enters the classroom runs to me to hug me. I lose my balance and fall. I pass out and come to lying on the floor with this student perched on my chest.   I am taken to the hospital by ambulance. I am not diagnosed with a concussion in the hospital, only told that my CAT scan and my MRI were clear.

Lesson # 3: CAT Scans and MRI's are often clear with concussions. These scans are not sensitive enough to show the microscopic damage that concussions can cause to the brain.
Not feeling well one week later, I was diagnosed by my primary care doctor with a concussion. I was told to rest and that I should be fine within two weeks.

Lesson #4: No one told me what "rest" means for the concussion patient. It means absolutely NO screens. Do not watch television, play on the computer, or check your phone.   Doing so may lengthen your recovery time. After two weeks, I was not okay. I was suffering from daily headaches, balance issues and a new, troubling symptom of increased stuttering and speech difficulties.

Lesson #5: There is no hard and fast timeline for healing from a concussion. If you break your leg, the doctor may have a timeline of how long it will take the bone to heal. There is no timeline for a concussion. Every brain is different. I began to

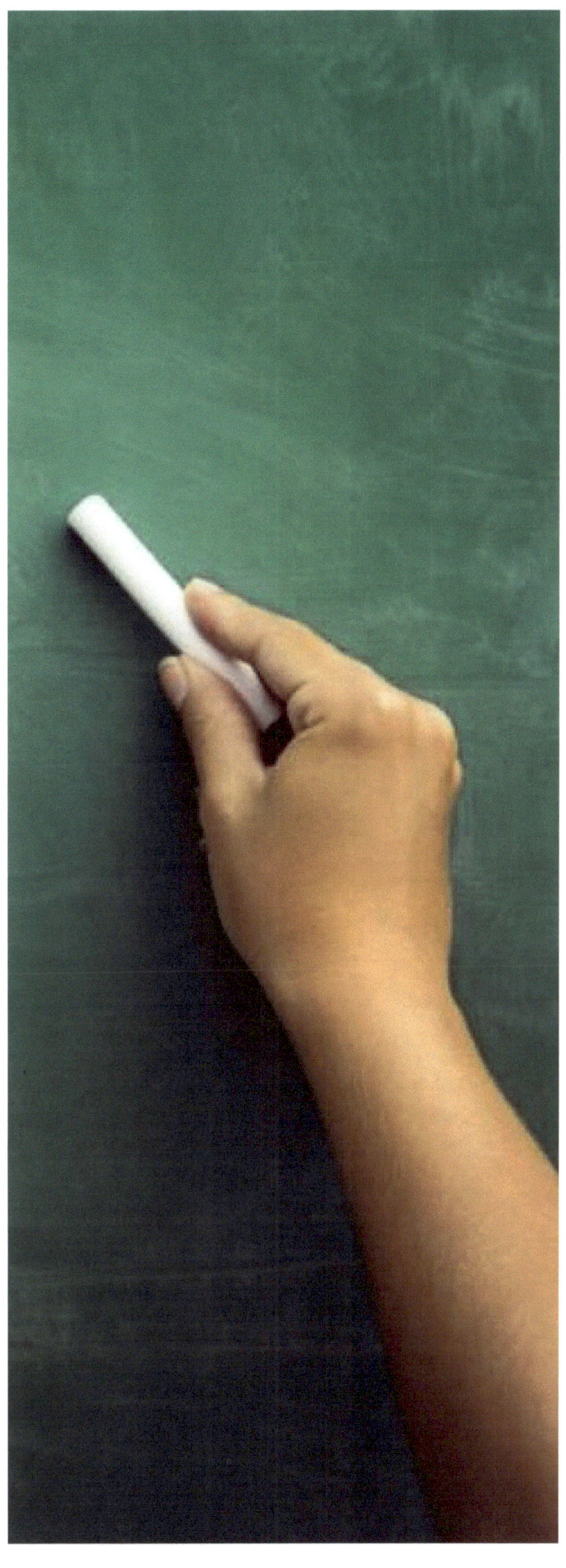

have spikes of extreme anxiety and feelings of depression. I blamed myself for these symptoms and was ashamed I felt this way.

Lesson# 6: Anxiety and depression are concomitant with concussion/brain injury. They are a part of the sequelae of symptoms, not a mental health disorder, pre-existing or otherwise. Doctors should be aware of this, but many are not. Three neurologists said that if I treated my mental health problems, all my other symptoms would resolve. I began to go from doctor to doctor searching for treatments. I saw doctors that were sympathetic but admitted they weren't sure what to do, doctors that maintained I had mental health issues only, doctors who were convinced that I was making up my symptoms. I eventually found a couple of competent doctors who helped me. I discovered that a combination of alternative therapies plus speech therapy worked for me. I love yoga, meditation and craniosacral therapy.

Lesson# 7: You must think out of the box. No one health care provider will have all the answers. Do not be afraid to try alternative therapies. Some people rave about acupuncture, although this did not work for me. I still battle many symptoms, headaches, speech difficulties, balance issues, cognitive confusion, but I am moving on.

Lesson# 8: Neuroplasticity - the brain can change and heal itself. I am not who or what I was before this injury, but my brain will continue to make new connections.   I have discovered a love for writing though I must do it in short sessions with frequent breaks. The doctors say I must adapt to my new normal.

Lesson # 9: This is perhaps the most important lesson of all – Never give up! It gets better. No matter how bad it is. It will get better.

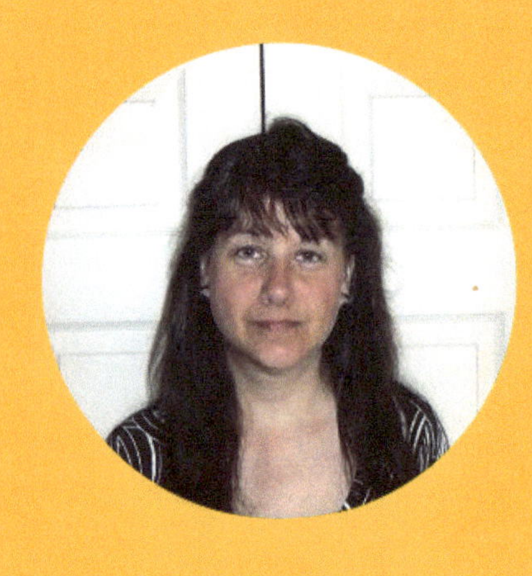

Meet Donna Cramer

Donna Cramer is a retired special education teacher who lives in Massachusetts. She worked with special needs students for over 20 years. She was injured at school. She stays busy doing yoga, pursuing therapies and education to further her healing from her injuries. Donna discovered a love for writing after her injury, particularly when she had difficulty expressing herself through speech. She wants everyone to know that there is always hope even though it may seem a distant, faraway glimmer there is still hope.

Bouncing Back

By Jeanette Drake

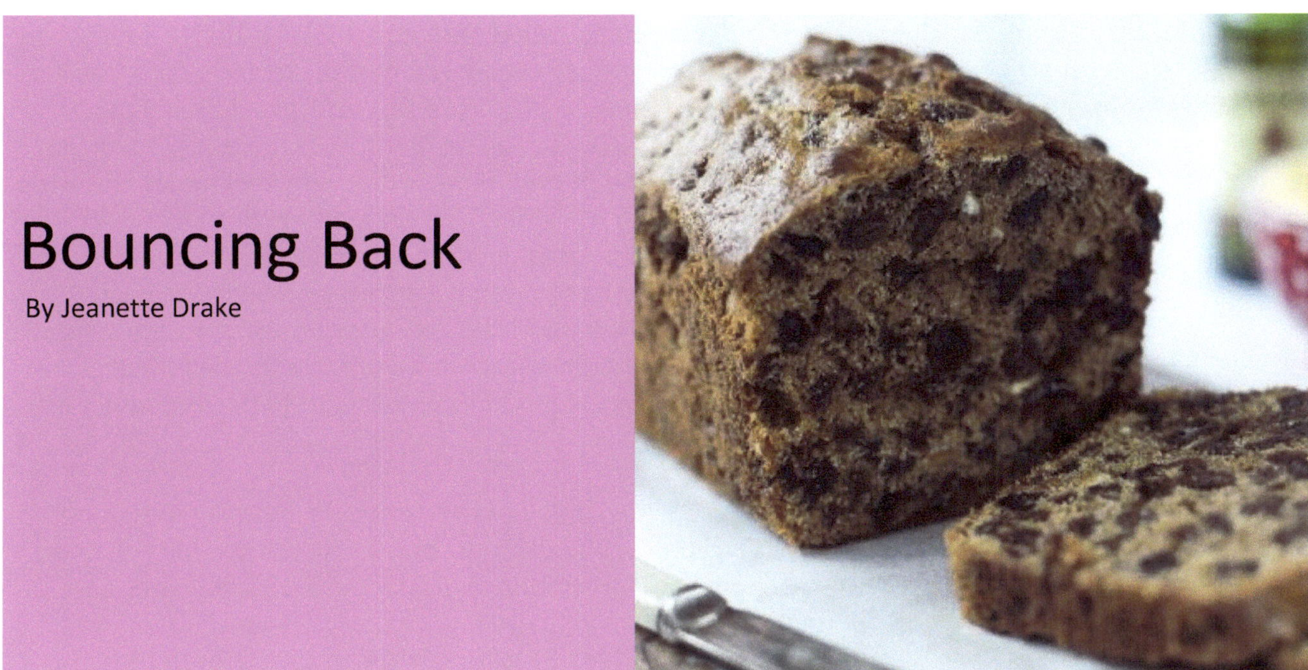

Two years ago, I was getting up during the night when I opened the bathroom door and slipped, that's all I can remember but from that moment my whole life changed. When I woke up, I did not know where I was There were tubes coming out of my neck and nose. I saw my husband and asked him where I was. In the most casual way you could imagine and quite typical of an Irishman, his first words were "How are ya doin'?"

He told me that I was in the hospital. During my time there my husband and daughters visited me a lot, my son and daughter-in-law also travelled long distances to see me. After a while, the doctor told me that I had a stroke. I do not remember much from being in hospital, though I do recall I recall the physio and speech and language therapist helping me a lot.

> *"I do not remember much from being in hospital, though I do recall I recall the physio and speech and language therapist helping me a lot."*

I spent two months there re-learning words and working on my speech and concentration. I could not put words together. My speech was definitely the most challenging aspect of my journey to recovery and I still find this exceedingly difficult now. I struggle to think of the words for what I want to say. Thankfully, people who know me understand this and have patience with me.

I was so happy when I left hospital to finally be back in my own home with my husband. After five or six months, I was asked to join a group by my social worker. The group was for people who are survivors of brain injuries. I joined this group to see if it would help with my memory and also to meet new people who have gone through similar experiences. The group is run by Acquired Brain Injury Ireland and is based only a few minutes' drive from my house -so I have no excuses not to show up!

Every Wednesday I go to the clubhouse. The clubhouse is called 'Bouncing Back.' I have been going there every week for six months now. There is also a group who attend on Thursdays. When I am there, I always make time to get my lunch. It feels lovely to be part of this group and I have met loads of new people here. We laugh a lot about doing yoga. We also go on day trips. One of my favorites was the day trip to see the Gardaí, the Irish word for the police. We got to try on the Gardaí uniforms, see their medals and their motorbikes. We do other activities like baking, reading, crosswords,

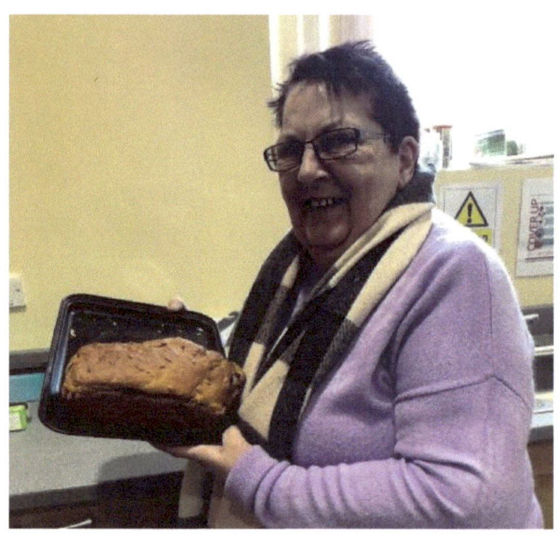

making Christmas decorations and much more. Marie and Vivian are the two rehabilitation assistants who help us by organizing all of the activities. In fact, as I am typing this, I have been told that we are starting a computer course soon – I am looking forward to this because I like computers.

I have done some baking with Kate recently. In the photo you can see I made a tea brack. This is my specialty and a traditional Irish food typically enjoyed with a good cuppa' tea. I actually made two tea bracks, but one was demolished by the others in the group before I took the photo! Today I will be busy planting sweet pepper seeds in the polytunnel.

Everyone in our group was given a vegetable to plant such as chili peppers, cauliflower, beetroot, tomatoes, broccoli, cabbage and lettuce. Even though it is raining outside (it always rains in Ireland!) we will still go out and prepare the polytunnel for planting. When the vegetables are fully grown, we will take them home and we also will share these with the Thursday group.

I am so grateful to all those who have helped me on my journey, in particular my family and the friends that I have made in this group!

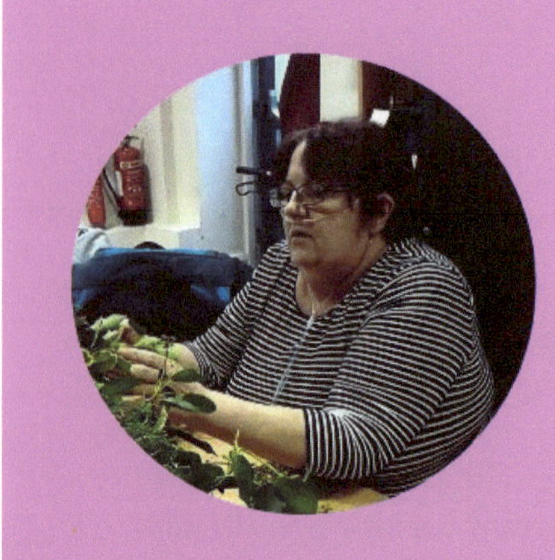

Meet Jeanette Drake

"Hi, my name is Jeanette Drake and I am a brain injury survivor from County Tipperary in Ireland. I did not know what a brain injury was until I had mine. Acquired Brain Injury Ireland is high profile organization that helps brain injury survivors with their rehabilitation. Without their help, I would not be where I am today. I was introduced to the HOPE magazine by Kate, a volunteer in the local group that I attend. It was interesting reading about other people's unique and individual stories, so, I wanted to use this as an opportunity to share my story with you."

Story Callout:

Navigating the GLOBAL PANDEMIC

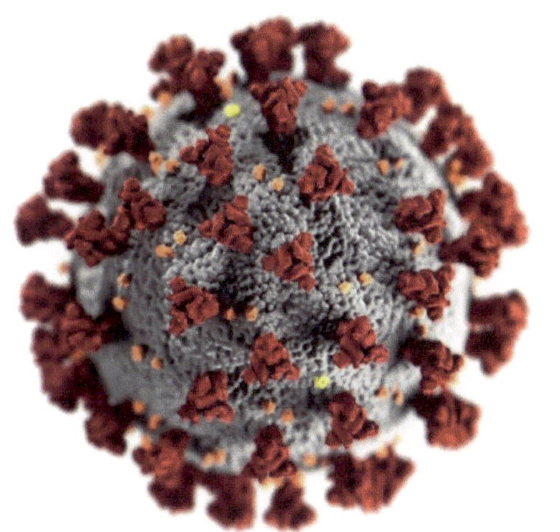

We are accepting stories for the Fall 2020 issue of HOPE Magazine about your experience navigating the pandemic as a survivor, family member or caregiver for someone with a brain injury.

These are challenging times indeed and your story can help others.

Our Fall 2020 issue of HOPE Magazine will be largely dedicated to this important topic.

Your Story has Value!

And now the details...

- We prefer an article length of 800-1,000 words. Longer or shorter pieces will be considered.
- When submitting, please include a photo or photos to be included with your piece.

Please email your submission to mystory@tbihopeandinspiration.com.

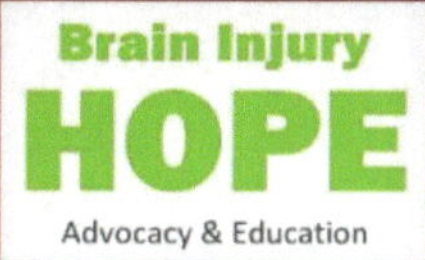

In A Moment

By Carol Nickerson-Goguen

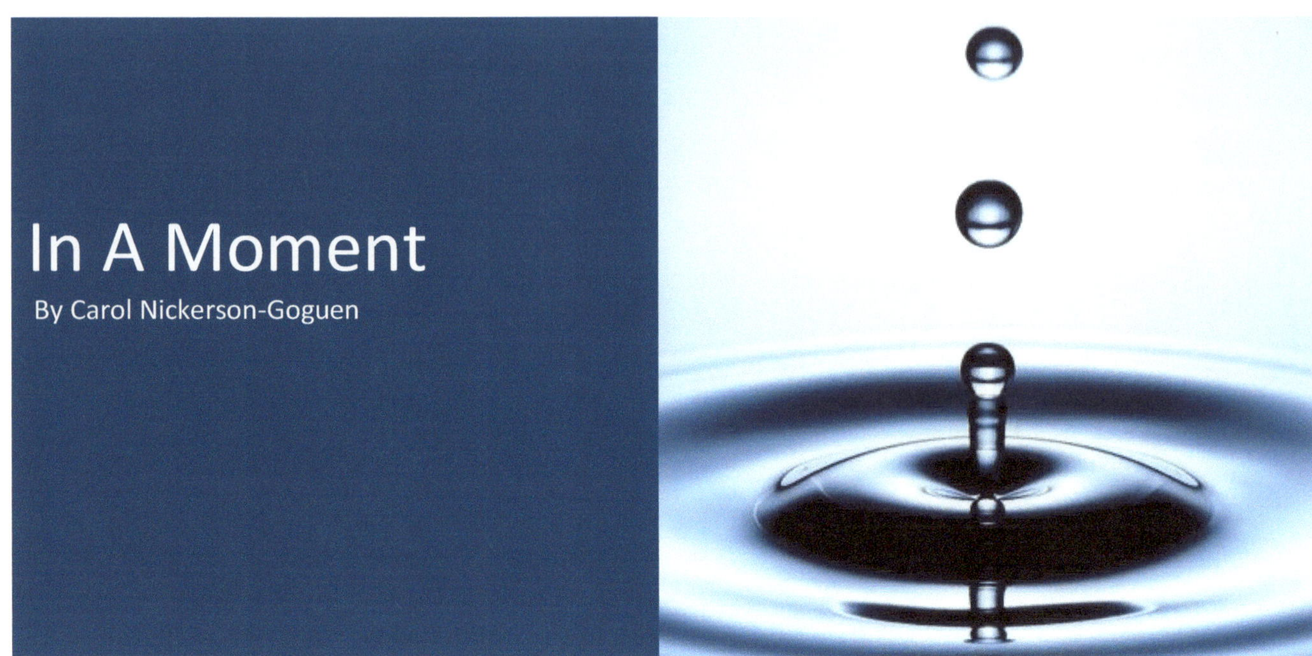

A moment was all that it took to absolve the life that I had lived for fifty-six years. On December 10, 2012, a slip on ice ended with the top of the head breaking the fall on ice covered concrete. I now jokingly say that the life of "Carol" almost made it to the end of the Mayan calendar. My car was parked at an office building facing a busy industrial street in Moncton, NB Canada. As a travelling Administrative Assistant for seven schools I left the office building on a work errand at 9:30 AM.

Walking towards my car, I noticed a car parked beside my car that was backing up. I stepped back to give the driver room, as I knew I was in his blind spot. As I approached the edge of the row, my left foot slipped on ice and I went flying in the air. I realized that I was falling so I dropped my purse and tucked my head into my chest to position myself to break my fall. However, I was in the air and could not keep my chin tucked. I tried to control my head as it whipped back, and everything went into slow motion. I could hear the hair swishing back in slow motion and I thought I could count the number of hairs in movement. It was surreal.

"With great difficulty, I opened my eyes and it was like I was seeing the earth for the very first Time. Everything was very bright even though it was a dark snowy day."

With great difficulty, I opened my eyes. It was like seeing the world for the very first time. Everything was very bright, even though it was a dark snowy day. The building that I had just exited was in total blackness from my newly lost left peripheral vision. I could see traffic moving in front of me on the boulevard as well as on the off ramp. From my right, I could see the traffic moving on the busy street. When I looked down, I saw the body falling and actually said out loud, "That's Carol."

I rushed to help the fallen person. Then I was suddenly back inside the body, I could feel the pain on the top of my head that already existed. I said out loud, "Thank you God for not letting me hit my head in the same place twice." Two years later, I still live in the fog, massive head pain, food is tasteless, and I cannot handle much light or noise. My left eye has a glaze over it that cannot be seen by doctors and it gets blurrier as the day goes on. I am always fatigued.

I was alone and made my way back into the office for help. My husband worked close by. I insisted that he was to take me to the hospital. I wanted to tell him of what I had just experienced. He knows I do not lie but he thought perhaps it was a dream, perhaps I was unconscious, but I told the emergency room doctor that I didn't black out and that I remembered everything vividly. Not telling him the whole experience would explain why he just sent me home to rest with a prescription for pain medication and no follow up or x-rays. I saw my family doctor two days later. He told me to stay home for a few weeks. He scheduled physiotherapy and prescribed another type of pain medication and ordered skull and neck x-rays. Then he was away for Christmas vacation.

Several days after Christmas I returned to the emergency room because the pain was unbearable. I was also nauseous, dizzy, and anxious. The doctor on call that night listened to my symptoms. He then ordered a CT scan for the next day and a referral to a specialist. It was the specialist who got to hear the entire experience. He put me off work for an additional month and set a follow up appointment in the spring.

Four months into this journey I found a closed Facebook support group, Brain Injury Awareness. I was lost and frantic and would post many questions to the other survivors and caretakers. They did not judge me, and they answered my pleas for help. They supported me and loved me. During these two years, I have worked hard at regaining my old self to return to work. I had six months of physiotherapy that involved pulled on my neck to align my spine.

Seven months into this journey, Workers Compensation sent me to their Workplace Recovery Centre for nine weeks. I was felt very privileged to attend as I was looking for as much help as I could get. I had a team that worked with me. I now had a doctor who changed pain and anti-depressant medications, and an Occupational Therapist, who also promoted Mindfulness. I did computer work alone in a dark room, having great difficulties preforming single tasks, while there were no attempts or schedule for multiple multi-tasking as my job required.

The Occupational Therapist got me walking without staggering within a few short days of being there by getting me to walk on my tip-toes and swinging my arms. I would practice this every night in my hotel room. I was very tempted to buy a pair of stiletto shoes!

I was reinstated back to my job and I did my best with my duties and practicing mindfulness. I did miss some days and time from work, due to head pain and being overwhelmed, anxious and nauseous, but I was determined to be the best I could be. I did the best that I could.

After being back at work for four weeks, I was called into the office of the Director of Finance, who, from a report of my supervisor, was told that they were not happy with my job performance. He told me he could see that I was struggling and was still in pain. He suggested that perhaps Workers Compensation had been too hasty recommending in my return. I had a doctor's appointment scheduled that morning and he recommended that I speak to my doctor about being taken off work for more recovery time.

I was devastated, knowing that I did my best. I was a crying mess when I got to my doctors' office. He seemed to agree with my employer and extended more time off. Workers Compensation did not agree and did not reopen my claim for compensation. I appealed their decision and it has taken over a year to have a hearing on this claim. Six weeks since the hearing, as I write this, I have yet to get a ruling on the appeal.

I was prescribed a multitude of various pain medication that did not touch the pain. Taking everything that my doctor prescribed for nineteen months, I realized through my own research that medications were actually slowing my healing progress. While on medication, I would sleep up to ten hours each night and another four hours each day. Depression and anxiety were getting worse, even though I was taking anti-depressants. I did not want life to continue as it was, and I asked my doctor how many pills I could take to end this life. He immediately called the emergency room physiatrist and an appointment was scheduled the next day.

I told the physiatrist everything I had experienced and how I was feeling emotionally and that I

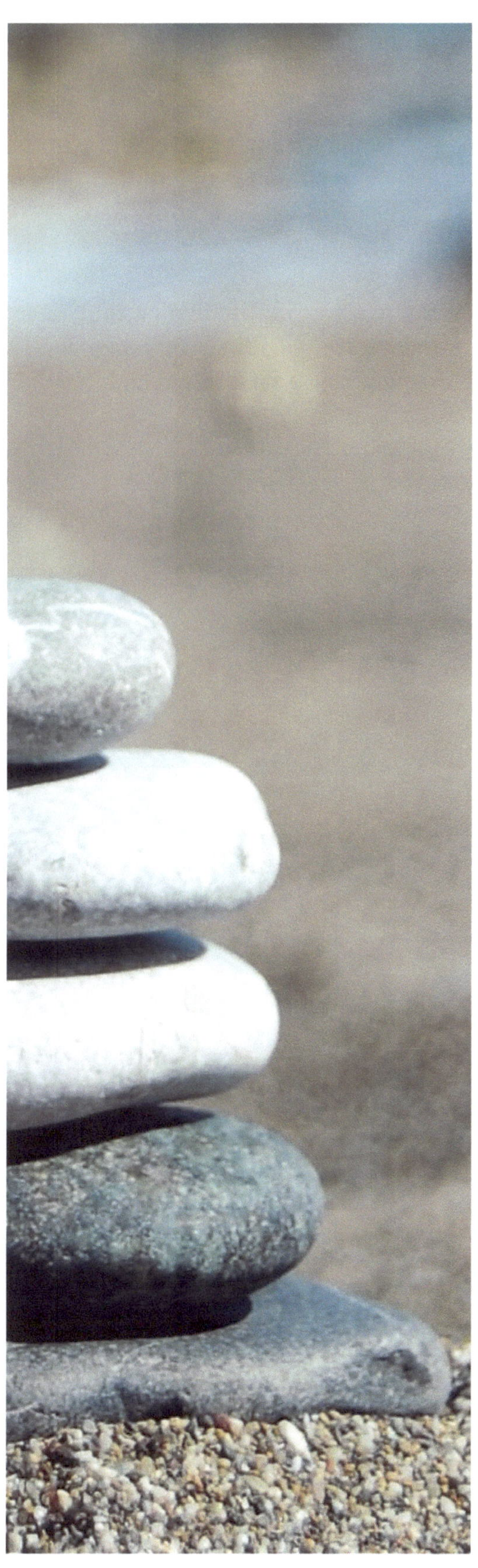

felt the medications were having an adverse effect on me and the new life I was left with. He told me I was absolutely within my right to stop medications. I did stop them without consulting my doctor on how to wean off them. That was a huge mistake as I was ill for two weeks. What my doctor referred to as Auditory Hallucinations were worse. I am greatly affected by lights and noise.

Shortly after I stopped the prescribed medications, I heard of the sports clinic at our local university and that they specialize in concussions. After a referral from my family doctor, I went to that clinic. The doctor I saw, knowing I did not want prescribed medications, recommended that I increase the Complex Vitamin B and Omega 3 that I was already taking and to add a high quantity of vitamin D.

I believe that my survival is due to on-line support groups. Knowing that I am not alone has been the biggest saving grace. I met other survivors on-line and had the privilege of meeting an incredibly special new friend from another province. She had her injury several years prior, and like many others, she fought a battle to return to work, only to be rejected. Since her injury, her daughter quit her job and enrolled in university to study to become a physiatrist. She has a great interest in Brain Injuries and became the provincial Brain Injury Association volunteer for New Brunswick.

On a very dark and stormy February day, she drove 140 kilometers to meet me and to accompany me to a local brain injury group meeting at the city hospital. She had created a provincial brain injury website and a closed Facebook support group, all the while studying and working part-time to pay her way through university. I met another new friend at the support group. She lives in a neighboring town and we communicate almost daily. I went to visit her this summer; well prepared with my google map. I got lost and was forty-two kilometers in the wrong direction.

I pulled into a rest station to gather myself from the overwhelmed and loss of confidence and intended on going home, but while driving towards home, it occurred to me where I made the mistake and headed in the direction of her home. I made it there, late, but we had a wonderful lunch and few precious hours together. That bonded our friendship.

It is hard to explain to someone the effects of Post Concussive Syndrome who has never had the experience. I once read that brain injuries affect one in every ten people, and those are only documented cases. I never knew of concussion symptoms prior to my fall or the devastating losses that come with it. Some doctors deny that there is anything wrong with the person who suffers a brain injury as the CT scan, EEG and skull x-rays all come back as normal. The patient is not able to explain it, not even to themselves. The devastation of the emotional hurt and loss, as family and friends vacate the life of a loved one, because they became suddenly different.

Post Concussive Syndrome entails a tremendous journey in attempts to navigate life in a painful fog. There is no "normal" in day-to-day living. In fact, most of my days are spent in a darkened, sound reduced room with ear plugs and sunglasses. How I wish this was just a bad dream and that one day, I would awaken pain and fog free.

I will continue to do the best that I can, and hope that in sharing my story, that someone may feel less alone.

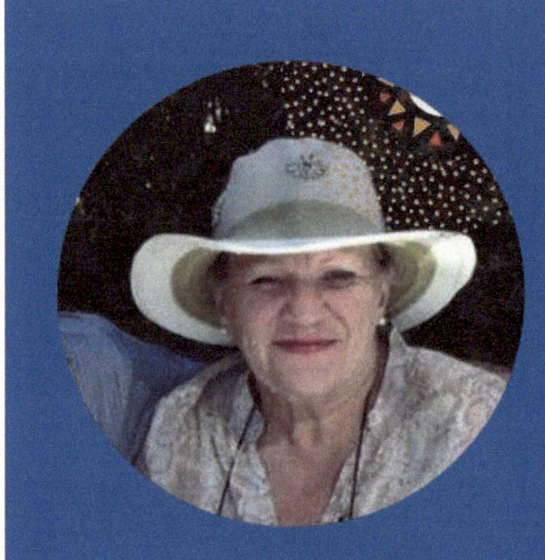

Meet Carol Nickerson-Goguen

Carol is a brain injury survivor from New Brunswick, Canada. Carol enjoys time spent with family and friends – especially those within the brain injury community. Carol is a strong advocate for all affected by brain injury and has shared her survivor experiences in her writing as well as through media interviews. A passionate writer, her poetry has been featured for publication by the World Poetry Movement. She hopes that her willingness to share will help others in their journey.

Living With Hope

By Patrick Brigham

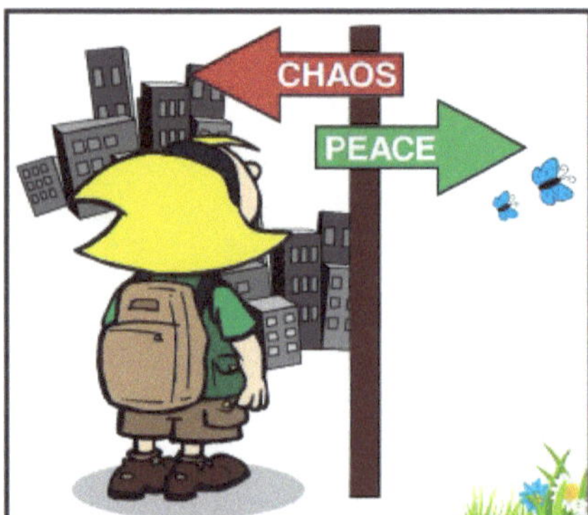

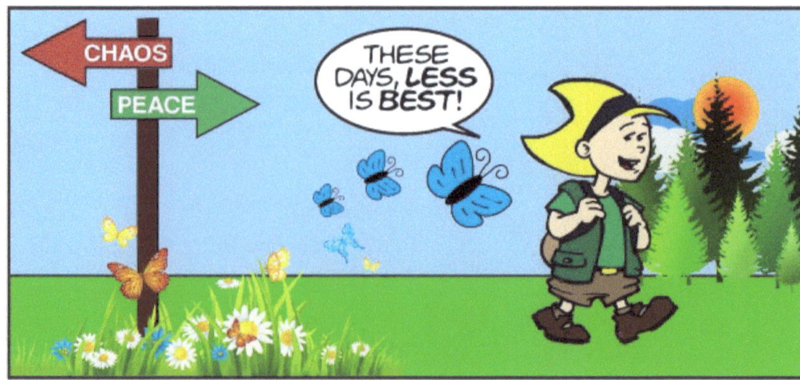

The World Has a
Brain Injury

By Lethan Candlish

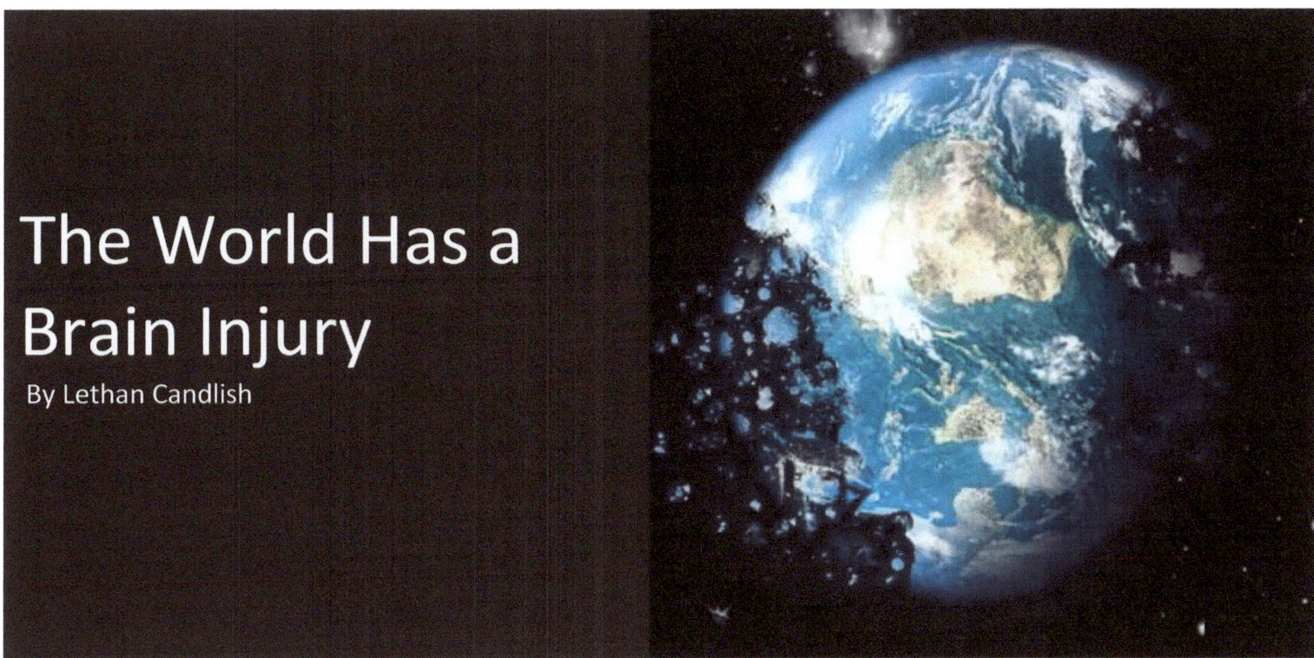

The world has a brain injury, though I don't mean this is the literal sense. As far as I know, Gaia isn't in a coma, but the current epidemic of Covid-19 has hit humanity in a manner that is questioning and dismantling many habits and institutions of modern society. Maybe it is not the world that has the injury, but humans that have been stuck hard and will require significant rehabilitation after the virus has been neutralized. I believe this process will in many ways mirror the introspective healing process that occurs after brain injury and recognizing these similarities will help humanity to find the most beneficial way to move into the future while better preparing for future catastrophic events.

> *"Maybe it is not the world that has the injury, but humans that have been stuck hard and will require significant rehabilitation after the virus has been neutralized."*

I use a simple method to demonstrate these similarities. Taking one stage of recovery at a time, I present what happens when recovering from brain injury and this if followed in the next paragraph by suggestions of the similarities in humanity's current crisis, suggesting how being aware of these similarities can assist us as we consider the road of recovery that is ahead.

For this comparison, I present the stages of recovery from brain injury as:

1) Initial Stabilization from the injury
2) Personal acknowledgement that an injury happened
3) Recognizing that a change is necessary and implementing new life patterns
4) Finding ways to maintain health

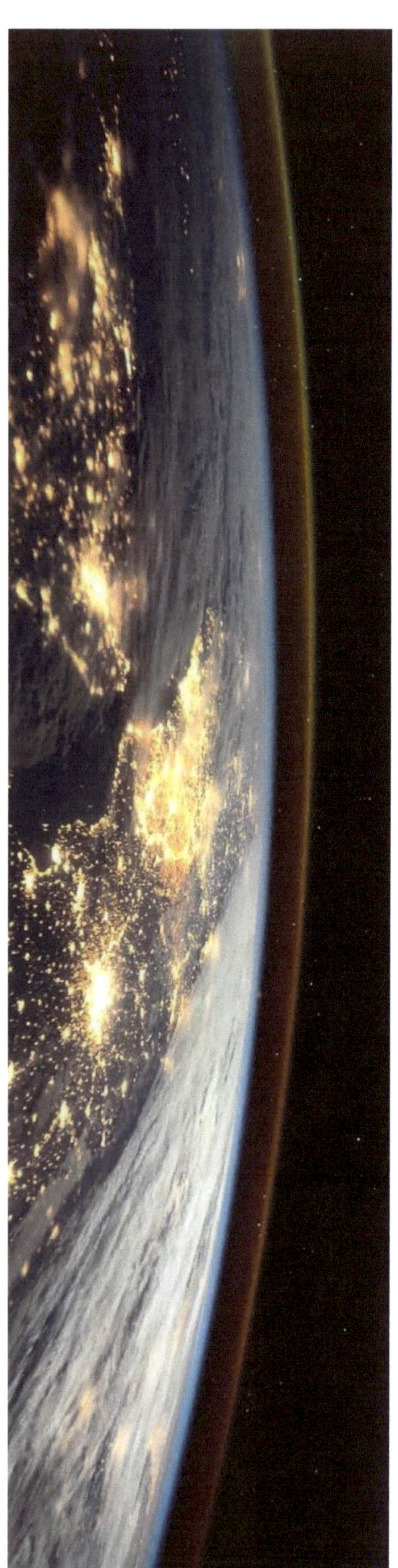

This list is not taken from medical literature, as I was not able to find any authoritative list that states a set of stages in the introspective recovery process. Rather, this list is created from a path I experienced over the first several years of my recovery from brain injury and I have recognized a similar process in stories I have heard and collected from other brain injury survivors.

Stabilization

First, the initial condition must be stabilized. In brain injury, this is when a survivor is rushed to the hospital and a medical staff works to ensure that life will continue to the next day. Thoughts and energies are focused on the immediate, on keeping the injured person breathing and the heart beating.

In our world situation, stabilization is what's going on now — the containment, social distancing, medical personal on the front lines of healing the disease, millions of necessary workers taking the risk to ensure that families can have food, electricity, and communication — these people are keeping the heart of humanity beating. As I write this article, it seems we are approaching the end of this initial stabilization period — perhaps still months away from fully moving to rehabilitation, but it seems that most countries have the initial plans of recovery in place and the panic has somewhat settled — we're going to live until tomorrow.

Acknowledging the Injury

The next stage is the survivor acknowledging the fact that the injury has irrevocably changed life. After brain injury, a survivor often wants to move on and forget about it, to put the injury in the rear view mirror and get back to things as before and letting the story become something told to friends. But the brain cannot so casually dismiss such an event. After brain injury there will be changes. These may be changes of attitude, of emotional patterns, personal preferences, habits, though processes, cognitive and physical skills, the exact combination will be is different for every survivor, but a person experiencing some set of changes is inevitable.

Acknowledging an injury means recognizing that change and learning how to adapt. In my recovery, an example of a change I have discovered is a tendency for my temper to flair suddenly and quickly burst into an uncontrolled rage — I need to recognize this about myself so that I can be aware when such anger might ignite and quickly put out the fires before anyone gets burned. If changes caused by brain injury are not recognized and synthesized into one's life, it will cause harm to the survivor and those emotionally close. Insisting that "things just need to go back to the way they were before" is a guaranteed cocktail of confusion, frustration, pain, and will quickly lead to disastrous consequences that often result in future injury.

In regard to the world's current situation, the event of the Coronavirus Pandemic will never be forgotten — as long as there is a hint of humanity that can share history this event will be in the textbooks. We acknowledge that the event happened — but we also need to recognize the change this is bringing to humanity. The situation is showing the fragility and underfunding of healthcare and education, the necessity of food and safety services, stripping away the false mantel of importance we have granted to so many jobs — and these are just a few of the insights the epidemic is highlighting. Social systems throughout the world are changing, and while the hope is that many of these changes will be temporary — that once the virus is contained, social systems will return to some relative norm — we cannot simply go back to "how things were before". This virus has hit the world hard and we must recognize what can never be the same.

Recognizing Need for Change and Creating New Life Habits

Once the situation has been stabilized and the injury acknowledged, a brain injury survivor must learn to adjust to the physical, cognitive, and emotional changes that have occurred. Adapting to these changes requires that a survivor create new life routines and habits that support the new way of living.

This does not mean that everything must change, but a survivor must be conscious of what habits need to be adjusted. Brain injury doesn't mean you cannot go to the gym, but perhaps you need to adjust your weight routine.

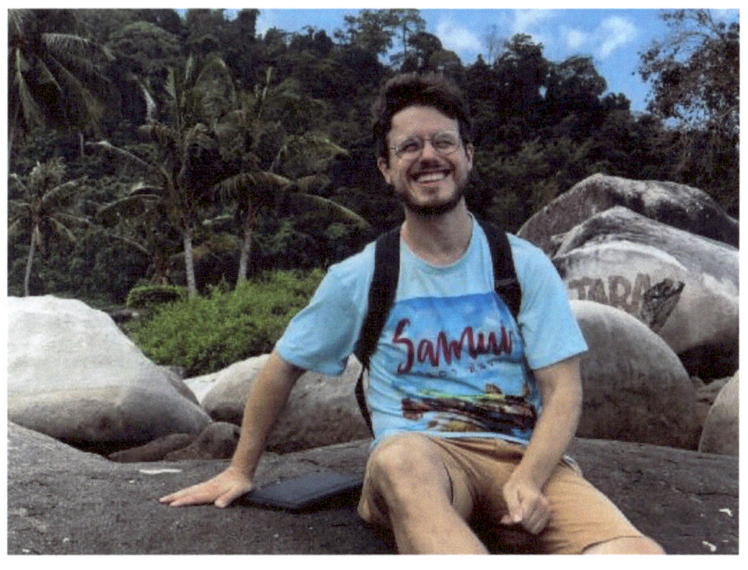

It doesn't mean you cannot see friends anymore but try going to a coffee shop instead of a bar. A survivor must approach the alteration of habits with an open mind that considers the reality of the effects of the injury — as discussed above — and create habits that support the new life conditions. This is best if done with the assistance of a team of medical and personal support persons that can offer suggestions. It is not an easy process, and some of these changes can go against social instincts that have been developed with a lifetime of repetition — yet recognizing and implementing these changes generally creates fewer frustrations and diminishes the risk of future injury.

A person may need to let go of previous habits, but allowing changes to occur and creating new habits can let a survivor flourish in ways previously never explored — personally, by allowing necessary changes to occur and accepting what must be, I had to give up my dreams of one career, but have found doors that opened to joys never considered prior to my accident. Being stuck on the idea of everything being the same as before leaves a survivor just that — stuck. Allowing life and habits to change will create new paths that encourages a survivor to continue forward in the journey of life.

Let us apply these same ideas to the Coronavirus Pandemic, because if we want humanity to continue into the next century, things have to change. We must find a balance between social welfare the profit motivation. Notice that now, in the midst of this pandemic, the greatest increase in stability has occurred when states, organizations, and brave individuals put social welfare ahead of immediate personal gain, and it has been this sort outreach that is helping to "flattened the curve."

The focus on international healing is inspiring, but it does not mean that humanity will not revert to the previous habits of personal gain once this crisis is contained. If we want to protect ourselves from some future injury of this scale — or worse — we need to embrace a new awareness of the necessity of social safety and education programs. The habits of the world can change — previous motivations may not work as guides anymore, but by consciously working together humans can find the safest and most rewarding path forward.

> "The focus on international healing is inspiring, but it does not mean that humanity will not revert to the previous habits of personal gain once this crisis is contained."

Finding Ways to Maintain Health

Maintaining a healthy lifestyle after brain injury is important for a brain injury survivor. Eating nutritious foods, finding time for some moderate exercise, and surrounding oneself with supportive persons will support to the brain's healing process. The logic is simple — if you provide the best upkeep and put the best nutrients into the body, the body will have more energy to heal. While this correlation is simple to state, it is not always easy to adhere to a healthy food and social diet after TBI. There can be physical limitations, confusion, depression, or any of the other effects from brain injury that can disrupt a plan for good health.

With dedication and by working with a support team, a healthy lifestyle will dramatically improve a survivor's healing, the mood improves, work quality can become mere consistent, and previous skills are relearned as the brain continues to heal. It is commonly said that the brain has "two years of optimal recovery", and after two years you are stuck with what you've still got. This is false. The body will continue to heal for as long as you let it, and by scheduling and maintaining a healthy lifestyle, a survivor will heal longer and more completely. The important thing is to create and maintain healthy patterns as soon as possible after the injury.

Creating and maintaining healthy patterns is what all of us — as the nations of the world — must do as we plan our future after the Corona Epidemic. It is likely that the majority of people in the world will survive this crisis, but it is inevitable that there will be deep and painful wounds that need to be healed — so many deaths, the pain of governments that were slow to react and initially failed citizens, an economy that has been stagnant for months — the aftereffects of this crisis will resonate in the world for years — decades — but we will heal. Yet we cannot view healing as a temporary state — it is important that we learn from this trauma and establish patterns and policies that support societal growth and health on a global scale — create healthy patterns so we can avoid a future calamity, or at least more adeptly respond when such a catastrophe arrives.

Final Thoughts

These are the parallels I see between the Coronavirus and brain injury. I do not pretend it is a perfect comparison, and there is overlapping of processes that occurs in the stages of recovery presented in this article — for example, where's the line between creating new habits and maintaining a healthy lifestyle — but the goal of this article is to encourage a conversation. This is how I anticipate the steps of international recovery that are ahead of us and what I hope governments around the world are considering as we navigate healing from this crisis. Humanity will be changed by this event — but as with brain injury, change does not mean an end. Instead, this is a mark on the timeline of humanity when we are forced to examine how we exist in the world — and there is potential in this moment for us accept a change that allows a healthier international community continue a beautiful growth into the infinity of the universe. Or we can remain stuck in the same patterns and hope another crisis doesn't hit.

The choice is ours.

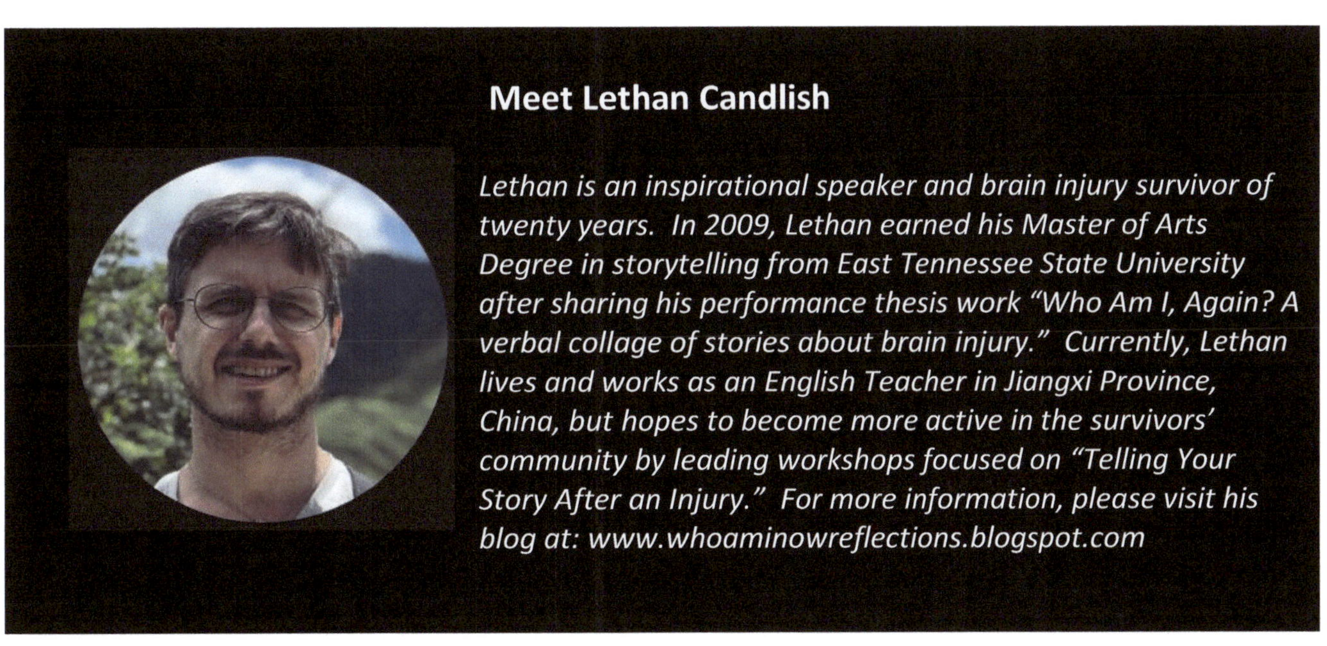

I'm not telling you it is going to be easy, I'm telling you it's going to be worth it.

-Unknown

Finding Fulfillment

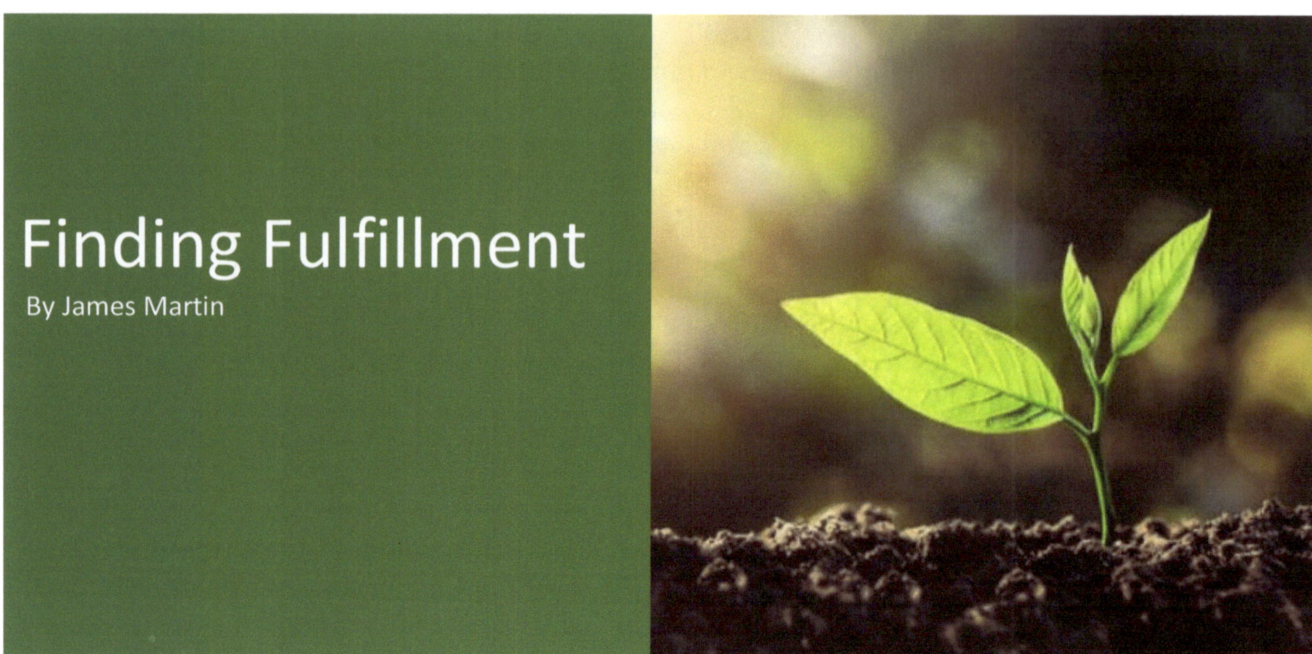

Over the past several years I have written about my experiences following having suffered a severe traumatic brain injury. For the most part, I expressed the desire to sustain hope in the face of tragedy. Recently, nearly nine years after my life changed by 180 degrees, I now realize that I am seeking fulfillment. Fortunately, for the better part of my adult life I enjoyed a successful professional career, was happily married, and watched my two children grow into successful and mature adults.

Then, it suddenly changed in ways I could never have imagined, physically, emotionally, and psychologically. In thinking about the transitions which I made over the past nine and a half years, I have taken great solace in Rabbi Harold Kushner's forward in "Man's Search for Meaning."

"After several years of seeking therapy, which was of enormous benefit, I am able to appreciate the contributions which I continue to make, albeit very different."

As he explained:

"The greatest task for any person is to find meaning in his or her life. Frankl saw three possible sources for meaning: in work (doing something significant), in love (caring for another person), and in courage during difficult times. Suffering in and of itself is meaningless; we give our suffering meaning by the way in which we respond to it…. Forces beyond your control can take away everything you possess except one thing, your freedom to choose how koi will respond to the situation. You cannot control what happens to you in life, but you can always control what you will feel and do about what happens to you."

After several years of seeking therapy, which was of enormous benefit, I am able to appreciate the contributions which I continue to make, albeit quite different. For example, I have volunteered at a local hospital one day per week for the past seven years. Although seemingly uneventful, to me, I cannot begin to explain nor express what my simple visits have meant to patients sitting idly by in a hospital bed, some for days to weeks, not knowing how or when they might recover. One of the units, RIO (Rehabilitation Institute of Oregon) is where I spent approximately ten days after having spent four weeks in two other hospitals following my TBI. The joy I experience when I can share with other patients in RIO, whether caused by a TBI, stroke, or other brain malady, not only my experience, but the opportunity to pass along even the slightest bit of hope, leaves me speechless.

As well, following receipt of a report from my treating neuropsychologist which stated, in part, that he had concerns that I may develop earlier than normal onset of dementia, I wandered into the local Alzheimer's Association and offered to volunteer. I was overwhelmed by the response, which has continued to this day, and now I find myself, among other things, being on the Board! A good portion of my role has been connecting the Association with local physicians in an effort to encourage referrals to the Alzheimer's Association for patients who have received that diagnosis, not for medical purposes but rather for the day to day realities of living with the disease. In addition, by connecting with the Oregon Medical Association, there have been numerous connections which benefit both parties.

In addition, there is a local nonprofit, Brain Injury Connections-NW, which provides support groups to the local community, both survivors and caregivers, for those who have experienced a brain injury, whether traumatic or acquired, and I find myself integrally involved in its operation as well, including but not limited to being an advisor to the Board.

The State of Oregon now requires that once an applicant passes the Bar Exam, that individual is required to have a mentor for approximately one year. Given my previous thirty years of practice experience, I have enjoyed the opportunity to pass along not only what I knew about practicing the type of law in which I was engaged, but as importantly who I knew, including several judges, both state and federal. My involvement in this program has kept me connected to the legal community in which I worked for so many years. And, in February 2019, after nearly fourteen months effort, I was successful in convincing both the plaintiff and defense trial lawyers to jointly sponsor a full day Continuing Legal Education (CLE) seminar concerning brain injury, traumatic or acquired. This effort was extremely fulfilling, both from a personal and professional perspective.

Moreover, having heard several times from many physicians who stated that what is good for the heart is good for the brain. Consequently, I have taken to exercising 6-7 days per week for approximately 1 - 1.5 hours and have never felt better! It has become, along with most other activities in which I engage on a daily basis, a ritual. Fortunately, it is a ritual I enjoy. Now, unforeseeably, we have been consumed with responding to Covid-19, the coronavirus which has essentially stopped everyone and everything in its tracks. So, for now, there is no gym available, the volunteer efforts to which I have been contributing have all but stopped, if not suspended indefinitely. My anticipation and hope is that there will be a return, but not to the "normal" which I have come to know. Consequently, I find solace in the following definition of Contentment:

Contentment is an awareness of sufficiency, a sense that we have enough, and we are enough. It is appreciating the simple gifts of life - friendship, books, a good laugh, a moment of beauty, a cool drink on a hot day. Being contented, we are free from the pull of greed and longing. We trust that life provides what we need when we need it. Contentment allows us to experience satisfaction with what is. We are fully present in this moment. Being contented does not obstruct our dreams or thwart our purpose. It is a place to stand and view the future with a peaceful heart and gratitude for all that is and all that is to come.

Consistent with the words of Rabbi Kushner, although I have no memory of the accident which caused by TBI, I believe that I now have some control over how I feel, and how I react, thereby exercising some influence over what happens to me in an ongoing manner.

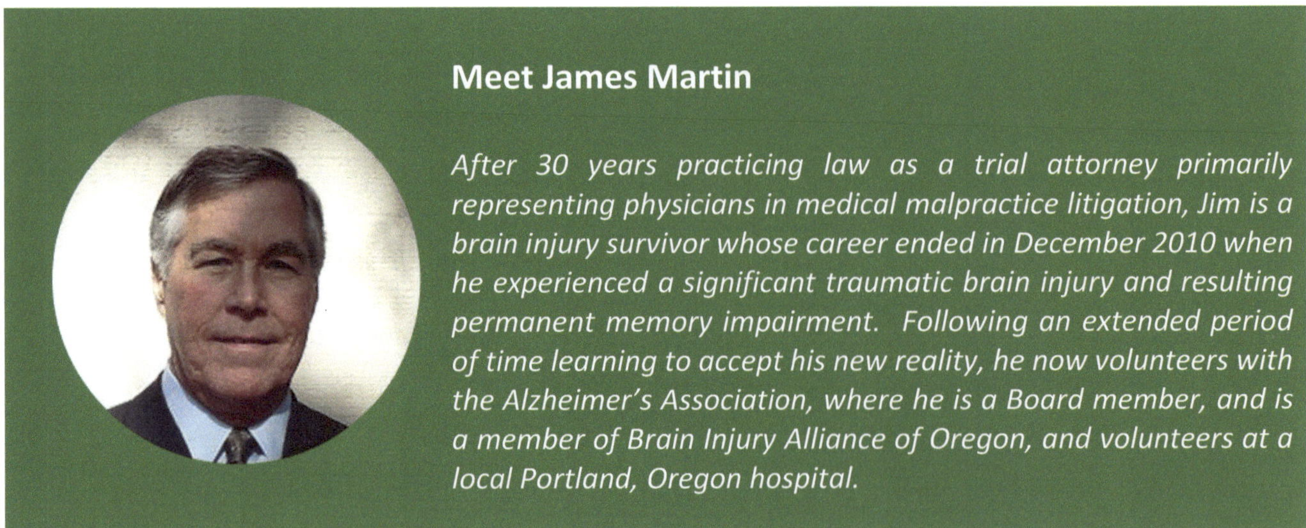

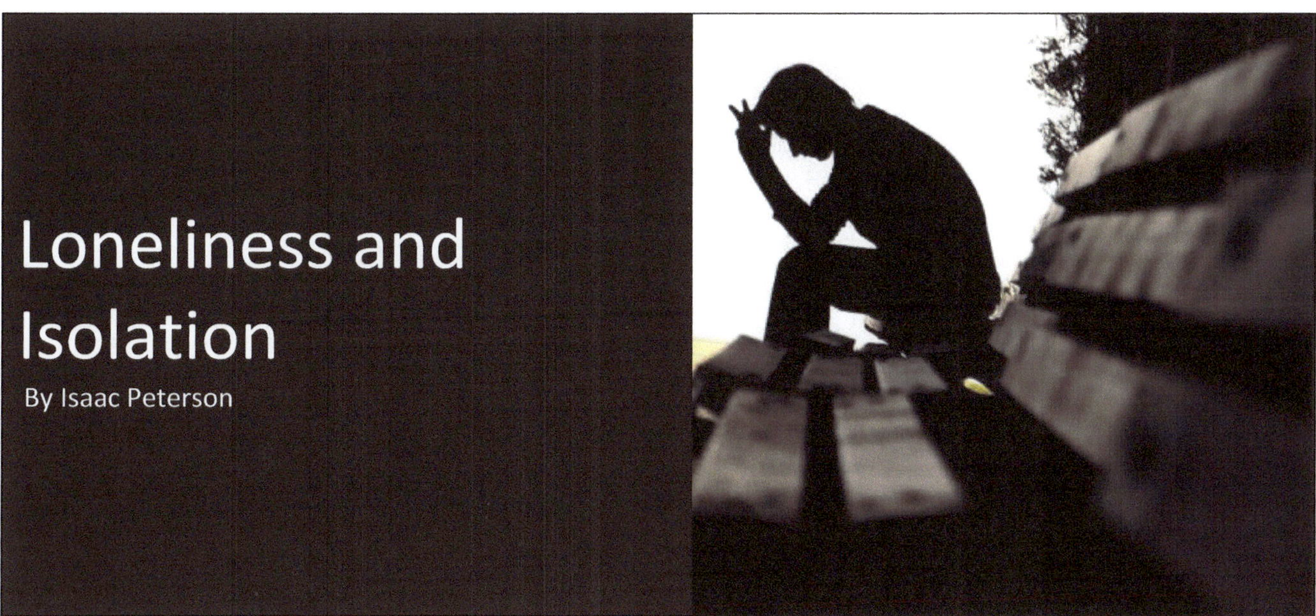

Loneliness and Isolation

By Isaac Peterson

Do you have a traumatic brain injury? If so, do you ever feel lonely and isolated, feelings many TBI survivors are forced to endure? I have a brain injury and have experienced those things, but to nowhere near the extent of others, who live with it all the time.

After experiencing a stroke and hospitalization in St. Paul, Minnesota I was involuntarily relocated to Tacoma, Washington. This was at the very end of 2016. I'm still here in Washington.

When I first arrived, I lived with my sister and brother-in-law. It was a lucky thing I at least had somewhere to go, since I only knew my sister and one other person, Nancy, a friend from college who also lived here. I only felt lonely and isolated a handful of times.

The first time was the worst, and it happened while I was in a houseful of people. I know it sounds goofy, to feel lonely in a crowd, but TBI survivors do not do a lot of things the way most other people without brain injuries do. The occasion was Christmas 2016, at my sister's house, and it was in the month following the stroke I had experienced. It was one of the most depressing days of my life.

> *"I know it sounds goofy, to feel lonely in a crowd, but TBI survivors do not do a lot of things the way most other people without brain injuries do."*

The place was jumping. There were a lot of people; at least it felt that way with my brand new brain injury and new aversion to crowds. And it was VERY LOUD. The sensory overload was excruciating. I felt very out of place with all the people filled with the holiday spirit of love and giving, while all I was filled with was the need to be somewhere quiet. And I was in a houseful of people who seemed to think a major stroke was something you can just bounce back from. I sat alone and feeling very lonely and isolated, surrounded by people.

I got through it somehow, but I don't know how.

After that, I only experienced that feeling of loneliness a handful of times. Here I was, in a place I had never been, and full of people whom I didn't know (yet). It was natural that I would have that lonely feeling, since it reflected the new reality I was living. I had come from a place where I was popular and well-known. It was a place where I had established myself as an accomplished journalist, but now I was in a place with a traumatic brain injury and no prospects or idea how, or even whether I would get back on track.

The lucky thing for me was that these times were few and did not last long. One of my saving graces was that I have had a lifelong love affair with books. I guess it was not completely true that I did not have any friends - I still had books. I was able to keep my mind occupied for hours at a time, sitting reading books, even though doctors had told me to avoid reading so soon after a stroke, as it would overstimulate my brain and make it have to work harder. I read and lost myself in the written word and characters who took the place of real, live, actual people and became my friends.

Another thing I did was just to go out and walk. Doctors had advised me not to do that either. But going out and being immersed in nature and fresh air seemed to be a real godsend and became a major part of my "new normal." I had been a dedicated walker my whole life. I did not have a driver's license until I was twenty-eight years old and haven't owned a car since about 1987. And one doctor told me he thought part of the reason I survived a major stroke was the physical shape I was in from walking. Walking figuratively saved my life again when I felt lonely and isolated. I know it sounds weird, overcoming loneliness by doing something where I was all by myself, but it worked.

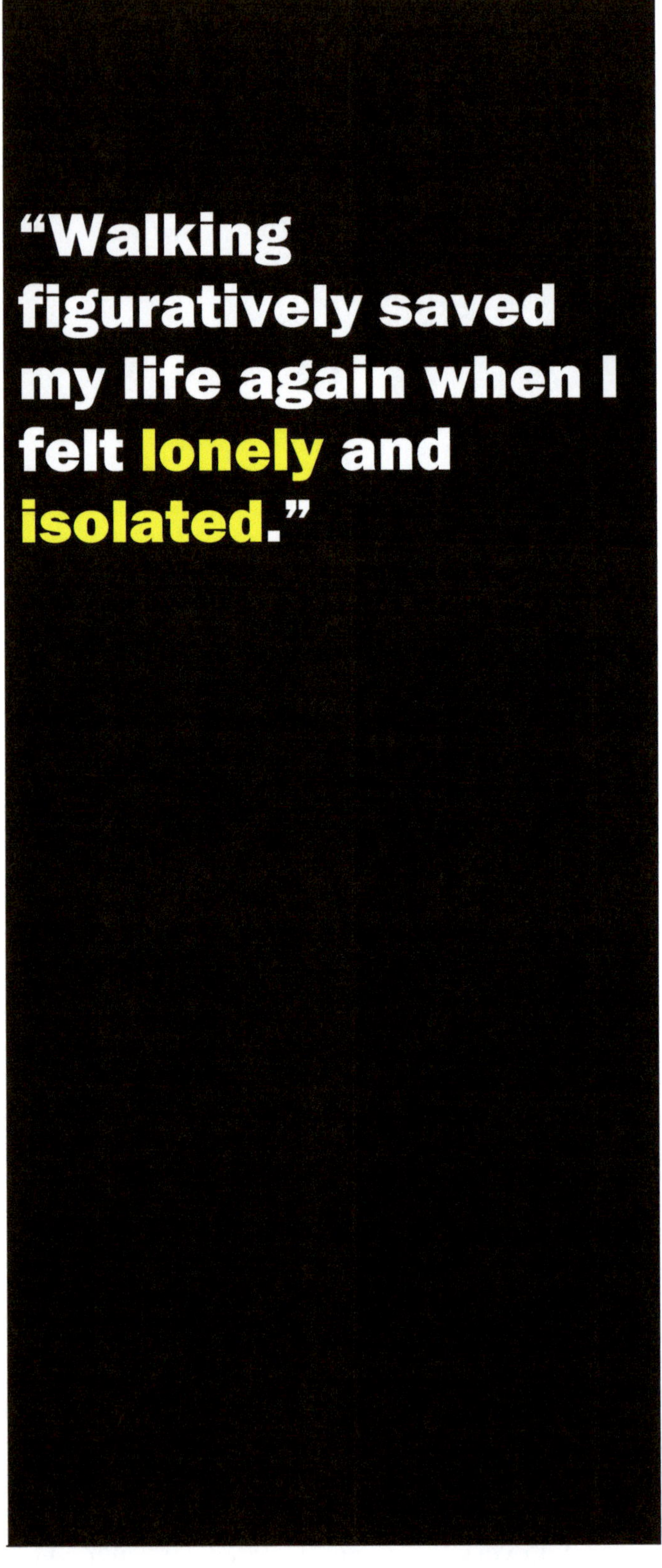

I know this is going to sound goofy and all 'new agey,' but I think it helped the feeling of loneliness, being outside and feeling a part of the universe and knowing I was part of something bigger than myself or anybody else, in a universe where everybody else and everything else also live. I did not feel so alone.

The few other times I felt alone my remedy was to just sleep. That took no effort since much of the time I had trouble staying awake anyway. I always felt better when I woke up. The move I made that went the furthest to helping with that feeling of isolation and being alone was joining the Brain Energy Support Team (BEST)TBI support group. There I was with other people who had the same feelings I had; it was a great place to meet and be around people who were all in the same boat.

It was the facilitator of the group who pointed me in the direction of being a blogger. I feel a great connection with my readers and have not felt truly alone since I resumed writing.

So there it is - how I navigated my way through loneliness and isolation. Your mileage will vary. Find the things that work for you.

And don't lose faith that things will get better!

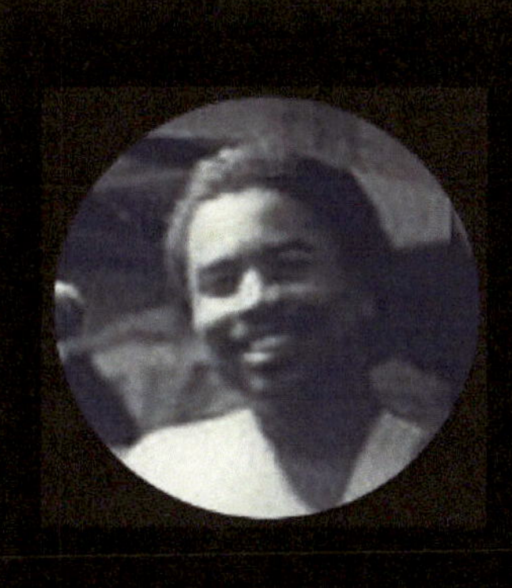

Meet Isaac Peterson

Isaac Peterson grew up on an Air Force base near Cheyenne, Wyoming. After graduating from the University of Wyoming, he embarked on a career as an award-winning investigative journalist and as a semi-professional musician in the Twin Cities, the place he called home on and off for 35 years. He also doesn't mind it at all if someone offers to pick up his restaurant tab.

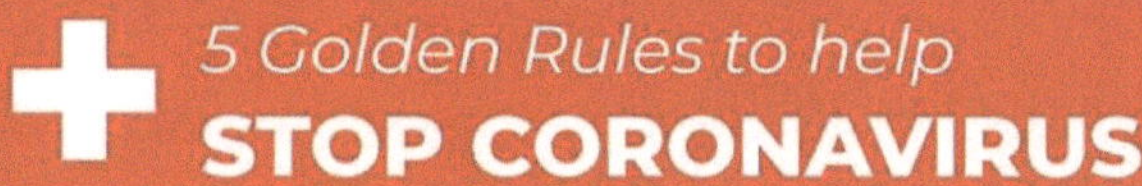

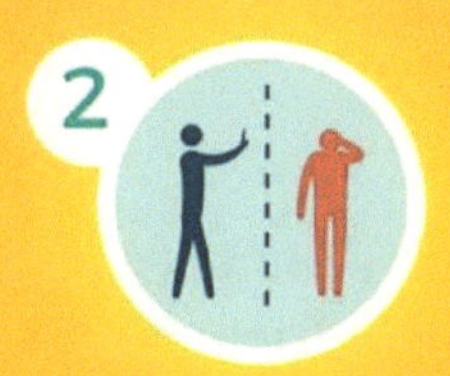

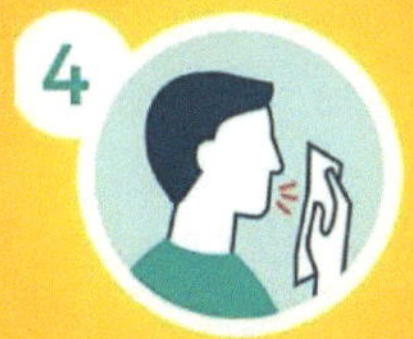

Drastic Change Again

By James Scott

I recently was honored to have a piece I wrote on acceptance featured in the Spring 2020 issue of Hope Magazine. In my writing I tried to express my deep gratitude for all the amazing help I've received throughout my BI recovery from a car crash on 7/4/06. Since I wrote *"Living Life on Life's Terms,"* something I never thought would happen has occurred - another drastic change. Only this time it's the way the world functions around me, not the way I function in the world that has changed. Call it a pandemic, national emergency, call it whatever you prefer, but the bottom line is that a lot of us have seen huge change in our daily lives.

Over the course of one's life, the only thing that seems to be constant or guaranteed is change. These transition periods, although a constant in life, can be distressing. While not necessarily limited to negative changes like loss or illness, these difficult periods, even after positive developments, can certainly be challenging. When we talk about loss, the first thing that comes to mind is death. Death is of course the ultimate loss, a singular event from which there is no possible return to a prior state.

> *"Over the course of one's life, the only thing that seems to be constant or guaranteed is change."*

As I always like to say when I feel like I'm pontificating, I can only offer my personal experience, although perhaps readers will relate: Post TBI I've felt an eerie calm from an expectation that after the crash, I would be insulated from additional traumatic events, or at least better prepared. Not that I would be immune from all the ills of ordinary humanism or never experience tragedy again, rather my handling of the situation would be exemplary.

In case you're wondering, this hunch has been proven inaccurate by the unease I've experienced living through this period. Don't get me wrong, I'm blessed that my friends and family are healthy and that I still have a job, but at the same time, the sudden change in the ways of the world has thrown me for a loop. As much as I try to remain positive and remind myself that "this too shall pass," the cunning trap of self-centered based pity is right at my doorstep during this period.

As I typed the term "self-centered based pity," the need for clarification was screaming at me from the screen! I admit self-centered may not be the best descriptor, so I'll clarify. In my now over ten years as a member of the Krempels Center, among the many helpful tools I've acquired, is the ability to identify faulty thinking. While I don't have the complete list of these logical errors or mistakes in thinking, common enough to have a fancy name, memorized, I poignantly remember one such error as being personalization. Perhaps I strongly identified with this particular error because I'd perfected making it?

Although self-pity, particularly when paired with "self-centered," brings to mind an individual with the mindset of, "I'm not much, but I'm all I think about." I certainly don't mean to infer that I'm an egomaniac. When I take a step back, this pattern of thinking is certainly understandable. Out of necessity, after my brain injury, there was a period where my world became quite small and hyper focused on "me." Early therapy was focused on assessing skills, identifying deficits, setting goals, and charting the progress I made. Often an unintended consequence of this intense period of reflection/analysis is the tendency to see the world as revolving around yourself. I've found that it takes work and a constant effort to break free of this mindset and simply join the stream of life.

To join the stream of life, to be another functioning part of the world, isn't that what I worked so hard in all those rehab sessions for? Maybe, but it isn't always an easy role to slide back into regardless of the progress made and time passed.

I hate making assumptions, but I have to think that any surprise that shakes the norms of the entire world such as this global pandemic causes widespread unease.

> **"I've found that it takes work and a constant effort to break free of this mindset and simply join the stream of life."**

Add to that the personal past experience of having our lives' derailed for brain injury survivors and it's no wonder that these may be stressful times.

Perhaps the most beneficial aspect of joining an amazing community-based day program like Krempels' Center is being a member of a group of survivors striving towards creating a new life after brain injury! None of us members are happy about the injury that made us eligible for membership, but Krempels' is an absolute blessing in our lives.

Like any transition, learning to and becoming comfortable with life with a brain injury can be challenging: At KC we accept each other where we're at in our journeys, sharing experience and strength through the telling of our stories. I can't help but see the parallels with the current global crisis and the need for feeling a part of a community that all of us have.

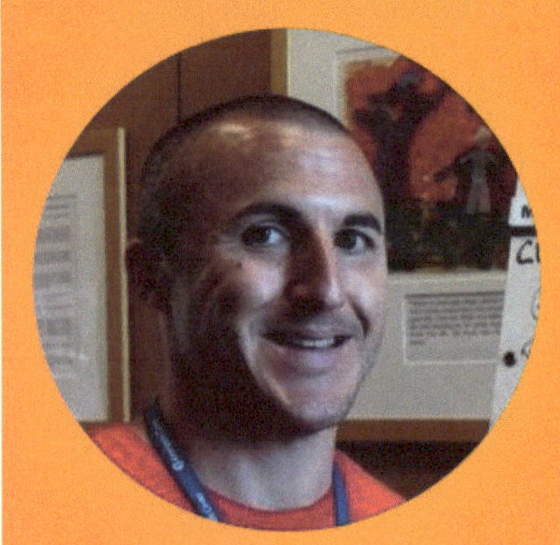

Meet James Scott

James sustained a TBI in a motor vehicle crash in July of 2006. Recognizing the cautionary value in his personal story, Jim first began speaking to students with KC's Community Education program. Jim has also worked with Northeast Rehabilitation Hospital's Think First National Injury Prevention Foundation. In 2012, Jim published a memoir titled More Than a Speed Bump: Life Before and After Traumatic Brain Injury.

Join our Facebook Family

What do almost 30,000 people from 60 countries and five continents all have in common? They are all members of our vibrant Facebook family at /TBIHopeandInspiration

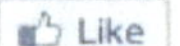

Amnesia

By Alonso Mendez

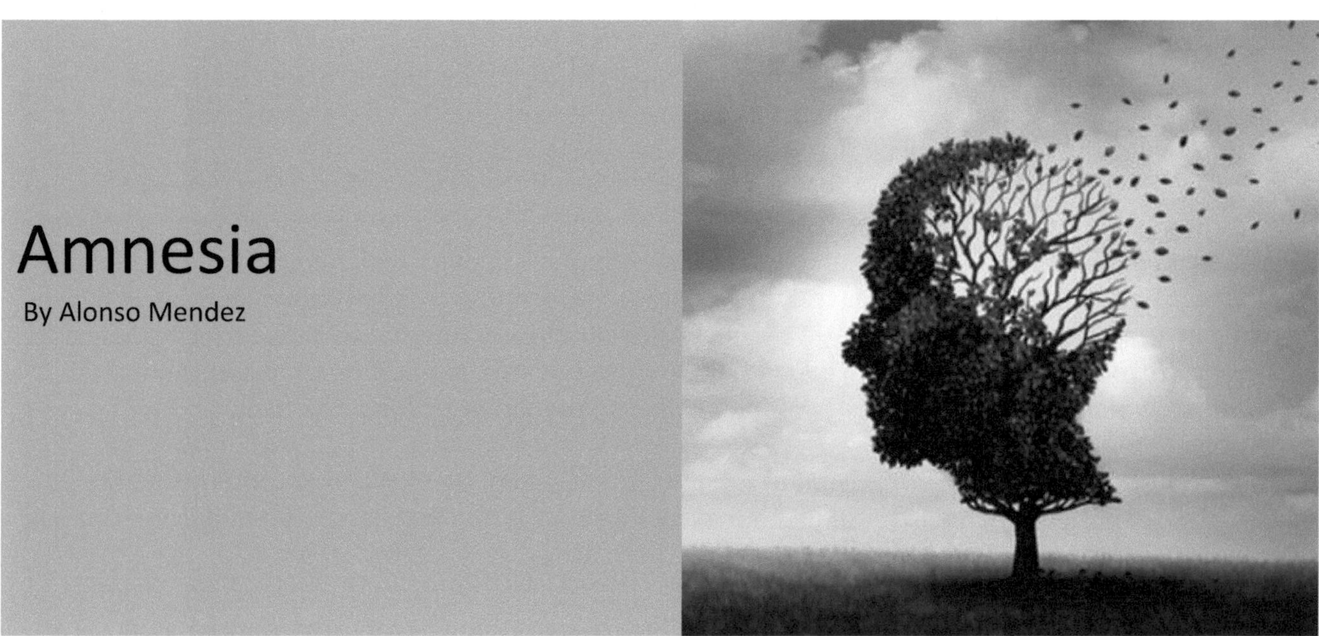

My name is Alonso Méndez, I live in México and I'm seventeen years old. I am passionate about psychology since I recovered from an accident that caused me a brain injury. That accident definitely changed my life. Since then I decided to get away from the vices and bad habits I use to have, in order to direct my life towards a direction in which I can help other people by supporting them psychologically.

I experienced what it is to suffer from this retrograde amnesia after suffering a traumatic brain injury on Sunday, June 2, 2019. To this day I have not been able to remember the moments before the accident, which involved alcohol and my vehicle. Due to the accident, I was unconscious for a week, later I was induced into a coma for another week. The first moments that I can remember are when I was hospitalized. I remember very little about it, some days my friends would visit me, on others, I did nothing but sleep and watch movies.

> *"To this day I have not been able to remember the moments before the accident, which involved alcohol and my vehicle."*

After a while, I returned to my house, and according to what my parents tell me, during the first weeks, by the time of happy hour I could no longer remember what I had done in the morning. When I was in a coma. I missed my girlfriend's graduation at that time, every day that she was going to see me I asked her when would her graduation be, to which she replied that I had already missed it. And the conversation would be repeated several times in the week, it seems that I wasn´t remembering anything she told me. She was visiting my house several times a week, but a few hours after she left, I would be asking my parents to invite her, arguing that I had not seen her in a long time. Psychological aftermaths?

It is something very sad for me to remember, but today I'm healthy and I have recovered from all the aftermaths of my accident and overcame all those risk factors I had as to the suffering of a post-traumatic disorder. Since many people can experience this type of experience in which they suffer psychological aftermaths due to an accident, it is important for other people to be aware that resilience is a skill that can be stimulated and enhanced (Porcar, 2015).   To enhance this ability, it is necessary to use our daily resources.

Such as planning our day with a time of relaxation, maintaining social contact, practicing sports (as long as the rehabilitation allows to), time for leisure activities, contact with nature, and relaxation techniques such as meditation. In general, the ideal is to return to the daily routine as soon as the clinical situation allows us (Porcar, 2015). These applications are referred to as the psychological first aids that we can apply to ourselves. This with the purpose mentioned before, to prevent those accidents in which we can be seriously injured, cause us psychological distress later.

It´s important for all of us to be prepared to overcome and accept these types of crises. If we don´t those crises would be capable to harm us, to make us lose hope and maybe spoil a bigger part of our life than what it should be.

We humans are like steel in that we are indestructible by everything except for our own oxide. It is important that we are prepared to be resilient and never lose hope. Because there always is, no matter how mentally or physically or emotionally hurt we are. We always have to stay strong!

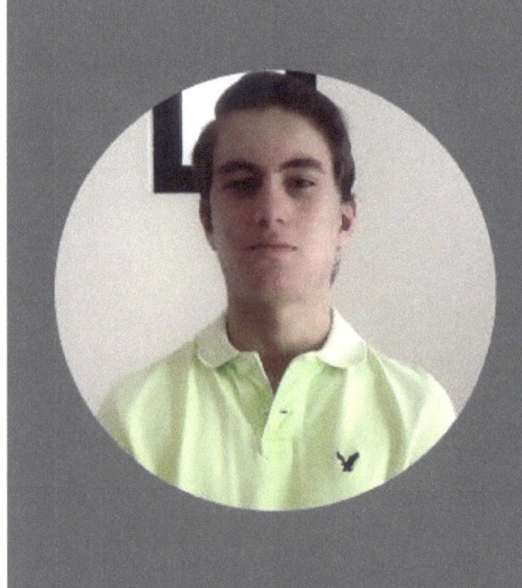

Meet Alonso Mendez

Alonso Mendez lives in San Luis Potosi, Mexico. He is a junior at Harkness Institute and plans to study psychology in college. He wants to learn ways to support and encourage people who are facing adversities such as the one he experienced on June 2nd,2019. He sustained a traumatic brain injury that provoked retrograde amnesia. His injury presented several risk factors and other psychological aftermaths such as post-traumatic stress disorder and vulnerability, which he has since overcome. Alonso recently completed online coursework in psychology, including an introduction to psychology, offered by the University of Toronto and psychological first aid course by the Autonomous University of Barcelona.

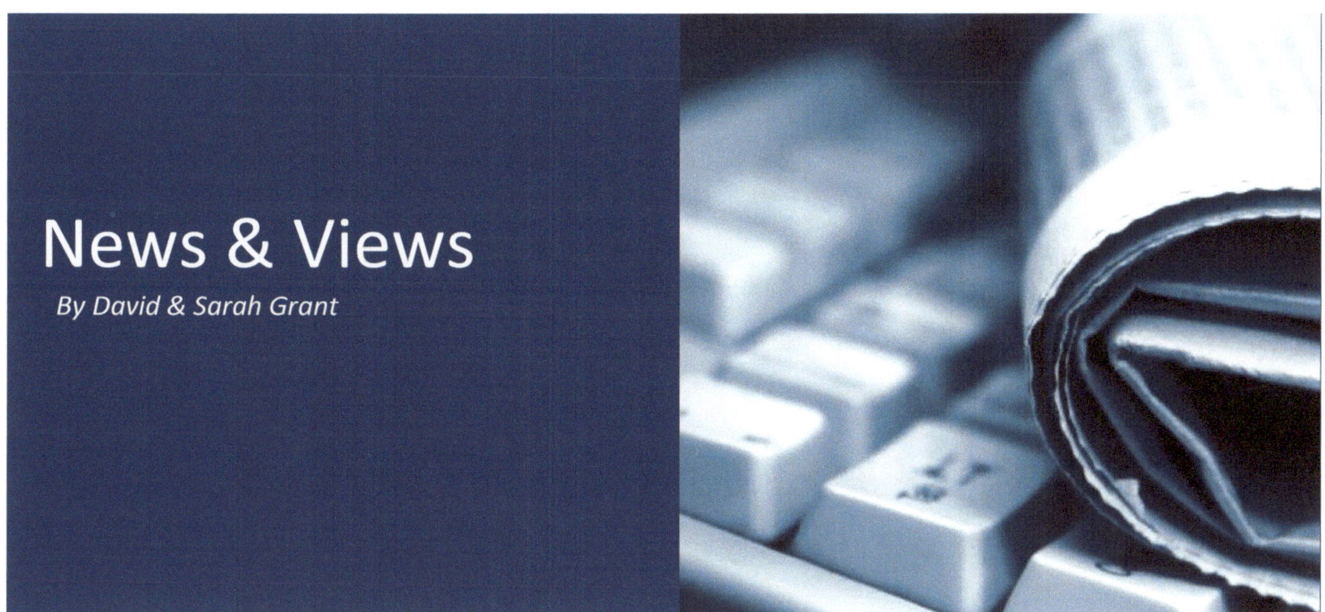

Since 2015, it has been our privilege to serve the brain injury community through the publication of HOPE Magazine. In the five+ years since HOPE Magazine began, we have had the opportunity to bring our readers hundreds of stories of hope and inspiration, stories that were penned by contributors all over the world.

Brain injury knows no geographic boundaries.

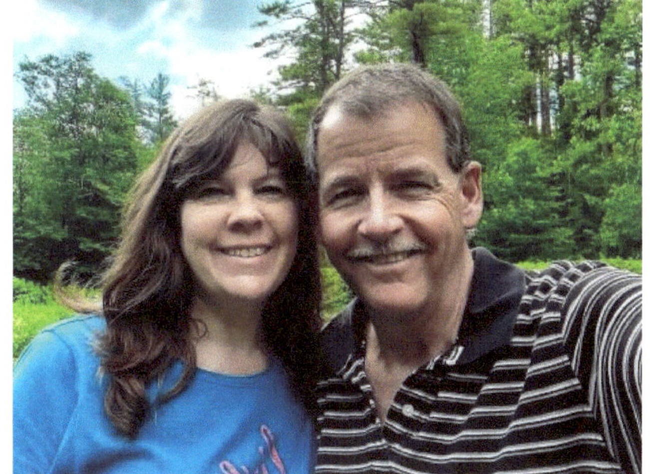

During these uncertain times, many of the traditional ways that survivors, caregivers, and others have found helpful have all but evaporated. Face-to-face support groups, a lifeline for so many, no longer meet. There is no realistic timeline for the return of these vital meetings.

Brain injury conferences, long a mainstay for professionals and survivors alike to get together to share knowledge and to simple "be" in the presence of others united for a common cause, have been cancelled – or replaced by virtual events.

There is no denying that the support landscape has changed dramatically. These days, there feels like a new urgency when we compile HOPE Magazine. For many, it is their only connection to others who walk the same path.

We remain committed to you – and wish you safety, peace, and hope during these times.

~ David & Sarah